T3-BIK-105

Benson/Phagan

Dental Hygiene: A Review for the National Board Examination

Barbara Benson, R.D.H., M.S.
Associate Professor and Coordinator
Dental Hygiene Program
William Rainey Harper College
Palatine, IL

Patricia Phagan, R.D.H., Ed. D.
Professor and Chairman
Dental Hygiene and Auxiliary Programs
Northwestern University Dental School
Chicago, IL

Quintessence Publishing Co., Inc. 1983
Chicago, Berlin, Rio de Janeiro and Tokyo

Library of Congress Cataloging in Publication Data

Benson, Barbara, 1939–
  Dental hygiene.

  Bibliography: p.
  1. Dental hygiene—Examinations, questions, etc.
I. Phagan, Patricia. II. Title.
RK60.5.B46 1983   617.6′01′076   83-16020
ISBN 0-86715-115-3

© 1983 by Quintessence Publishing Co., Inc., Chicago, Illinois. All rights
reserved.

This book or any part thereof must not be reproduced by any means or
without the written permission of the publisher.

Composition: Typographic Sales, St. Louis
Printing and binding: Edwards Brothers, Inc., Ann Arbor
Printed in U.S.A.

Contents

To our students, from whom we are always learning

Preface

Dental Hygiene is a profession. As such, it is an extensive compilation of basic science knowledge, which in turn builds a foundation for the acquisition of dental science knowledge. This special knowledge leads to the clinical arena, where all knowledge is assimilated in a plethora of ways in daily professional practice. The authors, having practiced as dental hygienists, having taught dental hygiene students, administered dental hygiene educational programs, and written questions for the National Board Dental Hygiene Examination, appreciate the complexities of the knowledge base of the profession.

This text is not, however, designed as a comprehensive work on dental hygiene. It is not everything you wanted to know about dental hygiene and more. It is not the authors' intention that you should use this text to learn the basics of dental hygiene.

This text is designed specifically as a review for the National Board Dental Hygiene Examination. The authors have organized the material to correspond to the examination. (Please refer to the outline provided in the Introduction and at the beginning of each chapter.) Each chapter corresponds to the various sections of the examination.

The National Board Examination does not have as its intent reexamination of the student on everything he or she has learned during the educational experience. The examination began in 1962 with a subject-oriented format. In 1969, the Committee on Dental Hygiene recommended replacing the four-part, subject-oriented examination with a comprehensive function-oriented examination, which included topics that correspond to the duties a dental hygienist would be expected to perform. After several years of development, the first function-oriented examination was administered at the March 1973 testing date.

Fifty-one jurisdictions currently recognize the National Board Dental Hygiene Examination as the written component of their licensure mechanism. These jurisdictions include all states within the United States, except Delaware and Alabama. Puerto Rico and the Virgin Islands also recognize the National Board Dental Hygiene Examination. The performance on the National Board is reported to the director of each dental hygiene program and to students who have done poorly, by subject. Subject classifications are Anatomy and Histology, Pharmacology, Periodontal Disease, Radiology, Dental Materials, Biochemistry and Nutrition, Dental Health education, Community Dental Health, Pathology, Microbiology, Instruments and Instrumentation, Physiology, and Plaque and Caries Control. The way in which the subjects are paired is subject to change from time to time.

Dental Hygiene is a dynamic profession. The study of the profession must adapt to the changes in the scope of the practice and be responsive to the needs of today's students. To this end, the authors have attempted to simulate the current National Board Dental Hygiene Examination as much as possible. The text is designed so that it may be used first as a "mock" examination, to be followed by use in an intensive preparation program for the actual examination. The authors administered the text as a mock examination to the 1982 and 1983 graduating dental hygiene classes of Northwestern University and William Rainey Harper College. Their suggestions and comments aided us immeasurably in the editing of the final text. For that input, the authors are very grateful.

Barbara Benson authored the Test-taking Strategies section within the Introduction as well as How to Use This Text and chapters 1, 4, 5, 7 and 8. Patricia Phagan wrote chapters 2, 3, 6 and 9. Realizing that the Public Health Section (chapter 9) is of a specialized nature, the authors enlisted the assistance of Ulana Kostiw, R.D.H., M.P.H., Assistant Professor, Northwestern University. Ms. Kostiw was recently named to the National Board Test Construction Committee for 1983. For her consultation, we would like to express our sincere gratitude.

You are now students. Whether you are also wives, husbands, parents, dental assistants, or in any other position in the work force is not relevant. You owe it to yourself to prepare for this examination in the most comprehensive way possible so as to realize your goals and the fruits of these years of labor, to become dental hygienists.

As educators, the authors have tried to assist you. As your imminent peers, we cheer you on.

The Authors

Introduction

The National Board Dental Hygiene Examination consists of 350 multiple choice test items. Between 10 and 20 percent of test items on any given test are in the "case problem" format. The examination content is divided into nine major sections. Each section poses questions in areas related to either background information, methodology, or armamentarium categories. Background information questions are those that cover foundation information in the sciences and dental hygiene therapy, and which are necessary for establishing an understanding for the techniques that you will need to use in daily practice. Questions related to methodology and armamentarium test the student's knowledge of performing a particular procedure, or demonstrate a skill and how to prepare the proper equipment and supplies for a specific procedure.

Outline

The specific content of each chapter is governed by the outline that follows. The functions treated in each section of the examination are followed by the number of questions relating to that function and the category in which the questions fall (i.e., A = background information; B = methodology or technique; C = armamentarium).

I. Performing Oral Inspection (52 questions total)
1. Extraoral inspection and charting (5 questions)
   a. observing external features (gait, skin, eyes, etc.) (3-A)
   b. palpation (1-A; 1-B)
2. Intraoral inspection and charting (30 questions)
   a. mucosal (8-A; 2-B)
   b. periodontium (6-A; 3-B)
   c. dental (4-A; 2-B; 1-C)
   d. occlusion (3-A; 1-B)
3. Identifying oral habits (3-A; 1-B)
4. Locating and identifying stain and deposits (7-A; 1-B; 1-C)
5. Evaluating oral hygiene status (3-A; 1-B)

II. Exposing and Processing Radiographs (46 questions total)

1. Exposing and evaluating (13 questions)
   a. intraoral radiographs (5-A; 4-B; 2-C)
   b. extraoral radiographs (2-A)
2. Radiation hygiene and safety (8-A; 6-B; 2-C)
3. Processing and mounting (2-A; 2-B; 1-C)
4. Recognizing normalities and abnormalities (12-A)

III. Providing Other Diagnostic Aids (32 questions total)

1. Obtaining medical and dental health histories (tests, vital signs, emotional status, etc.) (16-A; 2-B)
2. Preparing study casts (9 questions)
   a. taking impressions (3-A; 2-B; 2-C)
   b. pour, trim and mount (1-A; 1-B)
3. Clinical testing (thermal, vitalometer, percussion, transillumination, caries activity, cytologic smear, etc.) (3-A; 2-B)

IV. Performing Prophylaxis (43 questions total)

1. Scaling and root planing (12-A; 12-B; 6-C)
2. Soft tissue curettage (6-A; 3-B)
3. Polishing (coronal surfaces and appliances) (1-A; 2-B; 1-C)

V. Applying Topical Agents (17 questions total)

1. Caries preventive (7-A; 3-B; 1-C)
2. Anesthetic (2-A; 1-B)
3. Tooth desensitizing (2-A; 1-B)

VI. Providing Individual Oral Health Instruction (Including Nutrition and Plaque Control) (56 questions total)

1. Identifying needs for counseling (19-A; 5-B)
2. Planning instruction (13-A)
3. Providing instruction (8-B; 2-C)
4. Evaluating instruction (4-A; 5-B)

VII. Providing Supportive Treatment Services (46 questions total)

1. Asepsis and sterilization (6-A; 3-B; 2-C)
2. Pain control (9-A)
3. Polishing restorations and removing excess restorative materials (6-A; 2-B; 2-C)
4. Other supportive services (i.e., removing sutures, placing and removing surgical dressings and placing and removing temporary restorations) (8-A; 4-B; 4-C)

VIII. Assisting in Emergencies (28 questions total)

1. Recognizing potential for emergency situations (9-A)
2. Recognizing an emergency situation (8-A)
3. Providing emergency care (2-A; 7-B; 2-C)

IX. Participating in Community Health Activities (30 questions total)

1. Preliminary research (11 questions)
   a. identifying target population (1-A)
   b. identifying and measuring factors that influence oral health status (i.e., attitude, motivation, social, political and economic factors) (3-A; 3-B)
   c. establishing channels of communication to promote cooperation (1-A; 1-B)
   d. determining oral health needs (1-A; 1-B)
2. Project planning and operation (10 questions)
   a. defining project objectives (2-A; 1-B)
   b. developing project design (1-A; 1-B)
   c. identifying and gathering resources (1-B)
   d. selecting appropriate tools and media (1-A; 2-B)
   e. conducting activity (1-B)
3. Project evaluation (9 questions)
   a. gathering and analyzing project information (1-A; 2-B)
   b. comparing project results with preliminary data (1-A; 2-B)

c. determining the extent to which
   project objectives were achieved
   (2-A; 1-B)

Test-taking strategies

The National Board Dental Hygiene Examination is a multiple choice type of test. Each multiple choice item consists of a stem, which is either a problem, a question, or an incomplete statement, followed by options, of which only one is the correct answer and the others are distractors.

There is no substitute for content knowledge in answering test questions. However, test-taking strategies are simple common sense. And while it is true that test anxiety can influence your ability to read a question accurately, still you can increase your test-taking skills by analyzing types of multiple choice questions. The following are some simple strategies for analyzing such questions:

1. Be sure to read directions. For example, when reading the stem, "Which of the following are not true?" it may be helpful to underline the word not. In the stem, "Which one of the following is not true?" there are two key words in the direction. It would be wise to underline the words one and not because these two words give a strong clue to the answer.

2. Read the entire test item thoroughly. Consider the following test item:
   Dull instruments contribute to
   1. burnished calculus
   2. heavy handedness
   3. longer operating time
   4. slippage and trauma
   5. All of the above
   If you were reading too quickly, you might not have seen response number 5, which would be the correct answer.
   As you read each distractor, note the ones that seem correct. In this particular test item, since you can only have one correct choice as your answer, but there is more than one correct answer, number 5 would have to be your correct answer choice.

3. Some multiple choice questions seem more complicated than they really are. For example, let's examine a question from the section on pain control:

   Vasoconstrictors are contraindicated in patients who have
       (a) hyperthyroidism
       (b) cardiac arrhythmias
       (c) hypertension
       (d) prolonged bleeding
   1. (a), (b) and (c)
   2. (a), (c) and (d)

3. (b), (c) and (d)
4. All of the above
5. None of the above

Even if you are not sure of all of the distractors, you would probably know that vasoconstrictors are used in controlling bleeding; hence, they would <u>not</u> be contraindicated in this regard. (Hopefully, you would have underlined the word <u>contraindicated</u> in the stem.) So you would eliminate each response item that has (d) in it, as well as response item number 5, "All of the above." Your sheet would look like this.

1. (a), (b) and (c)
2. ~~(a), (c) and (d)~~
3. ~~(b), (c) and (d)~~
4. ~~All of the above~~
5. None of the above

Hence, you only have two possible choices remaining. And so your chances of selecting the correct answer are one out of two instead of one out of five.

In summary:

1. At all times, keep in mind the stated directions to individual questions.

2. Be alert to what the entire item is, not what you would like it to be.

3. Look for key words and underline them. Misreading and misinterpreting are a big source of errors.

4. Look for answers logically by eliminating those responses that you know cannot be correct. You will thus increase your chances of choosing the correct answer.

Again, test-taking strategies cannot make up for lack of preparation. They are merely an aid that may prove useful when you are actually taking the National Board Examination.

How to Use This Text

In order to gain maximum benefit from this book, you must view it as a learning instrument that should be part of your overall study plan for the National Board Dental Hygiene Examination. The following are suggested procedures for effectively using this text.

Phase I

1. First, remove the answer sheets. For the first time that you take the examination, you will stop at the end of each chapter and analyze your performance.

2. As you take the examination, mark the answers on one of the answer sheets provided. In addition, note the questions for which you do not know the answers or are unsure of the correct response.

3. At the end of the chapter, check your responses against the correct answers in the back of the book.

4. **Do not go on.** Review the chapter and its Recommended References again. For the questions you answered incorrectly, note the specific areas they represented, shown by combination number/letter codes (see example below). Interpret the code using the chart at the beginning of the chapter.

> 56. Which of the following is the best indi-
> **2bA** cator of gingival inflammation?
> ↑ 1. tissue color
> *code* 2. shape and form
> 3. consistency and tone
> 4. bleeding upon probing

For the example above, question 56 from chapter 1, the chart on page 15 decodes **2bA** as follows:

(2) about intraoral inspection
(b) of the periodontium
(A) background information

You should not simply memorize the answer to question 56, but *review* the background information about examining the periodontium, in the appropriate references.

Examine each wrongly answered question in the same manner. Cross-referencing between the charts and bold-face codes is a key to successful use of this book.

After you have completed all the other chapters and reviewed your weak areas, wait two weeks.

Phase II

Using a second answer sheet, take the entire examination again. Check your answers when you are half finished. Again, note down your weak **areas.** Then study and analyze these particular **areas.** Do the same thing on the second half of the examination. Wait three weeks.

Phase III

Now, simulate an examination environment. Note that there are more questions included here than are on the actual examination and that there is a predominance of combination answers (e.g., a, b and c; b, c and d; etc.). This examination may therefore take more time to complete than the National Board Examination. However, by now you should be familiar with this examination, so the time spent completing it should be about the same as for the actual examination. Allow yourself two three-hour blocks of time with no interruptions.

This time when you take the examination, mark your answers in the book. Note the amount of time that it takes you to complete the examination. At the end, evaluate your missed answers and again use the appropriate Recommended References to review those areas the question represents. The National Board will not ask a question that is not found in commonly used textbooks.

Finally, be sure to study old released examinations. These are very helpful in studying for the Boards, not only in terms of knowledge treated, but also in terms of familiarizing yourself with the format of the National Board Examination.

A major goal of this text is stimulation of thought and intensive study. In this regard, it would be beneficial if you were to formulate questions in areas for which you feel that you do not have a sufficient foundation. In this way, the director of your educational program may seek out those instructors responsible for that area of the curriculum and verbalize your concern. Such an approach, plus effective use of this text, perusal of the notes taken during your educational program, and study of previous released National Board Dental Hygiene Examinations should ensure successful completion of the examination.

Chapter 1

Performing Oral Inspection

Initial treatment planning is based on preliminary *oral inspection*. In addition to both extra- and intraoral inspection and charting, you must be able to make careful observations concerning your patient's oral habits and oral hygiene status. You must also be able to locate and identify stains and deposits. Time taken for this preliminary inspection will provide for better treatment later.

On the National Board Examination, there are 52 questions relating to the function of oral inspection. They are classified in the chart on the right according to the same three categories used in the actual examination: A=background information, B=methodology, and C=armamentarium. In every chapter, you will notice that under each question number there is a number and letter code. For example, for the first question in this chapter, the code is **2cA**. When you look at the chart to the right, you will notice that the number **2** refers to intraoral inspection and charting. The lower case letter **c** refers specifically to dental intraoral inspection and charting. And the upper case **A** means that this is a question concerning background information. If you miss this question, then you should review discussions of the *area* of intraoral inspection and charting as found in the Recommended References for this chapter. This coding system is used throughout the text, and you should always refer to the chapter chart to determine what areas—not specific *questions*—you need to study most for the National Board Examination.

Function	Questions and Categories
1. Extraoral inspection and charting	5 questions
a. observing external features	3-A
b. palpation	1-A; 1-B
2. Intraoral inspection and charting	30 questions
a. mucosal	8-A; 2-B
b. periodontium	6-A; 3-B
c. dental	4-A; 2-B; 1-C
d. occlusion	3-A; 1-B
3. Identifying oral habits	4 questions
3-A; 1-B
4. Locating and identifying stains and deposits	9 questions
7-A; 1-B; 1-C
5. Evaluating oral hygiene status	4 questions
3-A; 1-B

A=background information
B=methodology
C=armamentarium

Recommended References

Bhaskar, S. N. *Synopsis of oral pathology*. St. Louis: Mosby, 1981.

DuBrul, E. L. *Sicher's oral anatomy*. St. Louis: Mosby, 1980.

Pattison, G., and Pattison, A. *Periodontal instrumentation*. Reston, Va.: Reston Publishing, 1979.

Permar, D. *Oral embryology and microscopic anatomy*. Philadelphia: Lea & Febiger, 1977.

Wilkins, E. *Clinical practice of the dental hygienist*. Philadelphia: Lea & Febiger, 1983.

Woodall, I., et al. *Comprehensive dental hygiene care*. St. Louis: Mosby, 1980.

Questions

1.
2cA
Upon examining an 8-year-old patient, it was noted that the upper right second deciduous molar was missing due to extraction. Your recommendation would most likely be:
   1. There is no need for concern because the permanent bicuspid will be erupting within the year.
   2. There is no need for concern because the first permanent molar will drift into the area.
   3. The need for a space maintainer should be determined since the permanent bicuspid will not be erupting for some time.
   4. None of the above

2.
1bB
The anterior border of the mandible is examined extraorally by
   (a) bidigital compression of the tissues
   (b) circular movement on the soft tissues
   (c) beginning at the symphysis and moving posteriorly
   (d) beginning at the temporalis muscle and moving posteriorly
   1. (a), (b) and (c)
   2. (a), (c) and (d)
   3. (b), (c) and (d)
   4. All of the above
   5. None of the above

3.
2bA
Gingival pockets are defined as increased pocket depth due to
   1. apical migration of the junctional epithelium
   2. apical migration of junctional epithelium but coronal to the crest of the bone
   3. no more than a Class I furcation involvement
   4. proliferation of the gingival margin coronally with no apical migration of the junctional epithelium

4.
3A
Mouth breathing is an exacerbating factor in which of the following diseases?
   1. cancer
   2. gingivitis
   3. periodontosis
   4. gingival recession

5.
2dA
Radiographically, a tooth in traumatic occlusion may reveal
   (a) a widened periodontal ligament
   (b) vertical bone loss
   (c) root resorption
   (d) thickened lamina dura
   1. (a), (b) and (c)
   2. (a), (c) and (d)
   3. (b), (c) and (d)
   4. All of the above
   5. None of the above

6.
2aA
When examining the tongue, the operator notices the condition of "black hairy tongue." Which of the following papillae would most likely be affected?
   1. fungiform
   2. filiform
   3. circumvallate
   4. foliate

7.
2bB
A furcation involvement that allows the probe to extend *more* than 1 mm horizontally, but not completely through the furcation, is classified as
   1. Class I
   2. Class II
   3. Class III
   4. Class IV
   5. incipient

8. Nervousness may cause:

3A
1. nail biting
2. cheek biting
3. teeth clenching
4. attrition
5. All of the above

9. Which one of the following conditions

2aA is *not* thought to be related to emotional stress?
1. ANUG
2. leukoplakia
3. lichen planus
4. recurrent herpes lesions
5. recurrent aphthous ulcer

10. Tetracycline stain can be considered

4A which of the following?
1. endogenous
2. congenital
3. drug related
4. All of the above

11. Which of the following papillae are

2aA found on the lateral borders of the tongue?
1. foliate
2. filiform
3. fungiform
4. circumvallate

12. Tobacco stains can be considered

4A
(a) exogenous
(b) extrinsic
(c) intrinsic
(d) endogenous
1. (a), (b) and (c)
2. (a), (c) and (d)
3. (b), (c) and (d)
4. All of the above

13. All of the following conditions appear

2aA as white surface lesions of the oral mucosa *except*
1. candidiasis
2. chemical burn
3. geographic tongue
4. mucocele
5. leukoplakia

14. The temporomandibular joint is exam-

1bA ined extraorally by
(a) palpating bilaterally, placing the index fingers just anterior to the outer meatus of the ear
(b) asking the patient to slowly open and close several times
(c) asking the patient to perform right and left lateral movements with the teeth apart
(d) asking the patient to perform protrusive movement with the teeth together and then apart
1. (a), (b) and (c)
2. (a), (c) and (d)
3. (b), (c) and (d)
4. All of the above
5. None of the above

15. During an extraoral examination of the

1aA skin, the operator noted a macule. The following would be (an) example(s) of a macule:
(a) petechiae
(b) ecchymosis
(c) freckles
(d) melanosis
1. (a), (b) and (c)
2. (a), (c) and (d)
3. (b), (c) and (d)
4. All of the above
5. None of the above

16.
2aA
When the labial frenum pulls too tightly on the gingival tissues, it is thought to cause
1. ankyloglossia
2. cheek biting
3. gingival recession
4. linea alba

17.
2aA
The papillae of the tongue respond to various stimuli. Which of the following papillae respond to bitter stimuli only?
1. fungiform
2. filiform
3. circumvallate
4. foliate

18.
2dA
Occlusal problems can often be related to
(a) headaches
(b) sore muscles
(c) tooth sensitivity
(d) mobile teeth
1. (a), (b) and (c)
2. (a), (c) and (d)
3. (b), (c) and (d)
4. All of the above
5. None of the above

19.
2bA
Bleeding upon normal probing indicates
(a) that the epithelial lining has ulcerated
(b) that the pocket depth has deepened beyond the crest of the bone
(c) puncture of a healthy epithelial lining
(d) inflammation of the underlying connective tissues of the sulcus
(e) a deepened pocket depth
1. (a), (b) and (c)
2. (a), (d) and (e)
3. (b), (c) and (d)
4. All of the above
5. None of the above

20.
5B
A measurement of gingival inflammation is
1. the sulcular bleeding index
2. DMFS
3. CIS
4. deft

21.
4A
Submarginal calculus, as compared to supramarginal, has the following characteristics:
(a) It causes pocket formation
(b) It is dark brown, black, or green in color
(c) It is flatter in shape
(d) It is denser
1. (a), (b) and (c)
2. (a), (c) and (d)
3. (b), (c) and (d)
4. All of the above

22.
2aA
A rare, malignant lesion of the oral cavity that more frequently afflicts males than females is known as
1. hemangioma
2. melanoma
3. neurofibroma
4. lipoma

23.
1aA
When reviewing the health history, the operator noted spoon-shaped nails on the patient. This condition may possibly relate to
1. arthritis
2. cardiac disease
3. anemia
4. pulmonary edema

24.
2aA
Which one of the following lesions has the poorest prognosis?
1. leukoedema
2. Fordyce's granules
3. leukoplakia
4. melanoma
5. candidiasis

25. In horizontal bone loss, the crest of the
2bA alveolar process will be more than 1.5
mm from the cementoenamel junction. However, the configuration of
the loss will be parallel to the cementoenamel junction of each tooth.
1. The first statement is true; the second is false.
2. Both statements are true, but they
are unrelated.
3. Both statements are true and they
are related.
4. Both statements are false.

26. Which of the following is *not* a mea-
5A surement of oral hygiene index?
1. Massler PMA
2. Silness and Löe
3. OHI-S
4. PHP

27. Class II occlusion refers to the condi-
2dA tion where the
(a) mesiobuccal cusps of the maxillary molar and of the maxillary canine are mesial to mandibular landmarks
(b) mesiobuccal cusp of the maxillary molar aligns with the buccal groove molar
(c) maxillary canine rests between
the mandibular canine and the
first premolar
(d) mesiobuccal cusp of the maxillary molar is mesial to the
buccal groove of the lower first
molar by more than one-half
cusp
1. (a) and (b)
2. (a) and (c)
3. (a) and (d)
4. (b) and (c)
5. (c) and (d)

28. Vertical bone loss often occurs when
2bA the following conditions are present:
(a) The alveolar bone is thick.
(b) The alveolar bone is thin.
(c) Infrabony pockets are present.
(d) The base of the infrabony pocket is apical to the crest of the
bone.
1. (a), (b) and (c)
2. (a), (c) and (d)
3. (b), (c) and (d)
4. All of the above
5. None of the above

29. During an examination, an indication
3A of whether the patient has a bruxing
habit is an overdevelopment of which
muscle below?
1. temporalis
2. lateral pterygoid
3. masseter
4. buccinator
5. internal pterygoid

30. Evidence of nicotine stomatitis is often
2aA found in the
1. lingual tori
2. hard palate
3. plica fimbriata
4. sublingual caruncle

31. Submarginal calculus can be attached
4A to the root surface by
(a) scaling grooves
(b) cementum irregularities
(c) previous locations of Sharpey's
fibers
(d) calcified intracellular matrix
1. (a), (b) and (c)
2. (a), (c) and (d)
3. (b), (c) and (d)
4. All of the above
5. None of the above

32. When depressing the middle third of
2aB the dorsum of the tongue with a tongue blade and asking the patient to say "ah," you should see the
    1. posterior wall of the pharynx
    2. posterior pillars
    3. palatine tonsils
    4. anterior pillar
    5. All of the above

33. Green stain is most frequently found
4A in
    1. pipe smokers
    2. tea drinkers
    3. children
    4. older adults

34. The correct method for measuring the
2aB amount of attached gingiva is to use
    1. a probe
    2. a tongue blade
    3. a Nabers probe
    4. an explorer

35. Tori are overgrowths of bone often
2aA found on the hard palate and lingual areas. *Because* these growths often become cancerous in later life, they should be removed.
    1. Both statement and reason are correct and related.
    2. Both statement and reason are correct, but not related.
    3. The statement is correct, but the reason is not.
    4. The statement is not correct, but the reason is an accurate statement.
    5. Neither the statement nor the reason is correct.

36. Sodium flourescein is a stain that
5A 1. stains submarginal plaque orange
    2. is used with plaklite
    3. shows two shades of red
    4. has recently been removed from the market

37. Overjet refers to the
2dA 1. horizontal distance between the labial or lingual surface of the maxillary incisors and the facial surface of the lower incisors
    2. measured distance that the maxillary anterior teeth overlap the mandibular anterior teeth in a vertical plane
    3. measured distance the mandible moves forward in the condyle
    4. measured distance between the mandible and maxilla with the mandible in its most protrusive position

38. During an examination, it was noted
2aA that the throat was inflamed and sore. Treatment was contraindicated because
    (a) there was a danger of infecting the operator
    (b) multitudes of streptococci could possibly have been introduced into the bloodstream
    (c) if the patient had had a history of heart disease, subacute bacterial endocarditis could have resulted
    (d) the operator could easily have contracted herpes
    1. (a), (b) and (c)
    2. (a), (c) and (d)
    3. (b), (c) and (d)
    4. All of the above
    5. None of the above

39. The best means for detecting peri-
2bB odontal pockets is
    1. radiographic examination
    2. exploration with a pigtail (curved "cowhorn") explorer
    3. measurement with a probe
    4. testing for mobility

40. Upon examining a 6-year-old child,
2cA you would expect to find
    (a) four 6-year molars—3, 14, 19, 30
    (b) two permanent incisors—24, 25
    (c) three canines—6, 22, 27
    (d) two upper laterals—7, 10
    1. (a) and (b)
    2. (a) and (c)
    3. (a) and (d)
    4. (b) and (c)
    5. (c) and (d)

41. During exploration, the most fre-
4A quently missed areas of submarginal
    calculus are located
    (a) under the contact area
    (b) at line angles facially and lin-
        gually
    (c) at the bottom of buccal pock-
        ets
    (d) at the bottom of lingual pock-
        ets
    1. (a) and (b)
    2. (a) and (d)
    3. (b) and (c)
    4. (c) and (d)

42-47. According to C.V. Black's classifi-
2cC cation, which of the following classi-
    fications correspond to the diagrams
    below?
    1. Class I
    2. Class II
    3. Class III
    4. Class IV
    5. Class V

48. Dilated pupils could relate to which of
1aA the following?
    1. morphine
    2. barbituates
    3. amphetamines
    4. tranquilizers

49. Wharton's duct is associated with the
2aA 1. sublingual caruncle
    2. parotid gland
    3. buccal mucosa
    4. linea alba

50. Instruments for detecting submarginal
4C calculus include
    1. explorers
    2. probes
    3. radiographs
    4. air syringe, mirror, and light
    5. All of the above

51. Upon examining the dentition, an inci-
2cB sor is tested for pulp vitality. The fol-
    lowing procedure is indicated:
    (a) Check for the presence of a
        pacemaker.
    (b) Place the tester on the middle
        third of the crown of a single-
        rooted tooth.
    (c) Keep the teeth moist
    (d) Start the rheostat at 5.
    1. (a) and (b)
    2. (a) and (c)
    3. (a) and (d)
    4. (b) and (c)
    5. (c) and (d)

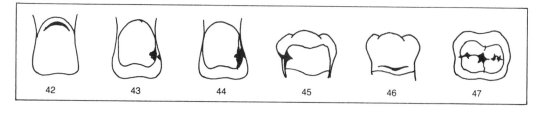

42   43   44   45   46   47

52. The OHI-S index includes how many
5A teeth?
   1. 8
   2. 6
   3. 4
   4. 10

53. The palatine uvula is located
2aA 1. near the palatal raphe
   2. near the palatine foveae
   3. in the soft palate
   4. on the median palatal raphe

54. When the mandible is held in the most
2dB posterior position, with the teeth together, and maintained without external forces pushing it back, this is
   referred to as
   1. malocclusion
   2. functional occlusion
   3. working occlusion
   4. centric occlusion

55. The predominant crystalline salt in cal-
4A culus is
   1. brushite
   2. whitlockite
   3. octocalcium phosphate
   4. hydroxyapatite

56. Which of the following is the best indi-
2bA cator of gingival inflammation?
   1. tissue color
   2. shape and form
   3. consistency and tone
   4. bleeding upon probing

57. Mobile teeth are best examined by
3B 1. two tongue blades
   2. an explorer and a curette
   3. the index finger and the thumb
   4. a mirror handle and a probe han-
      dle

58. The following is true when probing the
2bB interproximal area:
   (a) The area beneath the "col"
       must be probed facially and
       lingually.
   (b) The probings beneath the con-
       tact area will overlap for the
       mesial-facial and mesial-lingual
       areas.
   (c) The probe will angle into the
       interproximal area.
   (d) The probe will be angled paral-
       lel with the long axis of the
       tooth.
   1. (a), (b) and (c)
   2. (a), (c) and (d)
   3. (b), (c) and (d)
   4. All of the above

59. A soft, bluish, fluctuant mass that does
2aA not empty on pressure and is located in
   the anterior floor of the mouth is most
   likely to be
   1. a cavernous hemangioma
   2. a major salivary gland tumor
   3. mucocele
   4. a minor salivary gland tumor
   5. a ranula

60. Extrinsic exogenous stain normally can
4B be removed by
   (a) dry brushing with a tooth-
       brush
   (b) rubber cup polishing with
       pumice
   (c) scaling
   (d) ultrasonic scaling
   1. (a), (b) and (c)
   2. (a), (b) and (d)
   3. (a), (c) and (d)
   4. (b), (c) and (d)
   5. All of the above

61.
2aA
When examining the floor of the mouth, the operator notes an extremely short lingual frenum. This could cause which of the following conditions?
1. xerostomia
2. ankyloglossia
3. sublingual caruncle
4. plica lingualis

62.
5A
Which of the following disclosing solutions differentiate between old and newly formed plaque?
(a) FD & C Red No. 3
(b) Basin Fuschin
(c) FD & C Blue No. 1
(d) FD & C Green No. 3
1. (a) and (b)
2. (a) and (c)
3. (b) and (c)
4. (b) and (d)

63.
2bA
To establish a diagnosis of periodontitis, the following must be present:
(a) bleeding
(b) mobility
(c) probing beyond the cementoenamel junction
(d) plaque
1. (a) and (b)
2. (a) and (c)
3. (b) and (c)
4. (c) and (d)
5. None of the above

64.
4A
Which of the following ingredients in dentifrices has been reported to cause a brown/black stain?
1. sodium fluoride
2. acidulated phosphate fluoride
3. stannous fluoride
4. strontium chloride

65.
2cC
The choice of instrument for the detection of pit and fissure caries is a
1. sickle scaler
2. probe
3. shepard's crook (#23)
4. pigtail (curved "cowhorn")

Chapter 2

Exposing and Processing Radiographs

An important facet of daily operation for the clinical dental hygienist is exposing, processing, and interpreting radiographs. You have to be concerned not only with techniques in processing and mounting, but also with recognizing what is normal or abnormal on a radiograph. In addition, it is extremely important that you be aware of radiation safety at all times—to protect both your patient and yourself.

On the National Board Dental Hygiene Examination there are 46 questions devoted to the field of *radiography*. These questions are subdivided as shown in the chart to the right.

Function	Questions and Categories
1. Exposing and evaluating	13 questions
a. intraoral radiographs	5-A; 4-B; 2-C
b. extraoral radiographs	2-A
2. Radiation hygiene and safety	16 questions 8-A; 6-B; 2-C
3. Processing and mounting	5 questions 2-A; 2-B; 1-C
4. Recognizing normalities and abnormalities	12 questions - A

A=background information
B=methodology
C=armamentarium

Recommended References

Eastman Kodak Co. *X-Rays in dentistry*. Rochester: New York, 1977.

Frommer, H. K. *Radiology for dental auxiliaries*. 2nd ed. St. Louis: C. V. Mosby, 1978.

Kasle, M. J. *An atlas of dental radiographic anatomy*. Philadelphia: W. B. Saunders. 1977.

Langlais. R., and Kasle, M. J., *Intra-oral Radiographic Interpretation*. Vol. 1. Philadelphia: W. B. Saunders, 1978.

O'Brien, R. C. *Dental radiography: an introduction for dental hygienists and assistants*. 4th ed. Philadelphia: W. B. Saunders, 1982.

Wuehrmann, A. K., and Mason-Hing, L. R. *Dental radiology*. 4th ed. St. Louis: C. V. Mosby, 1977.

Questions

1.
1aA Which of the following statements best describes leakage radiation? It is that
1. radiation produced when primary rays strike matter.
2. radiation produced when electrons strike the target of the anode.
3. primary radiation from the tube housing, which does not pass through the useful beam aperture.
4. excess radiation escaping from a faulty X-ray tube.

2.
1aC The electrode from which electrons are emitted in the X-ray tube is the
1. anode
2. cathode
3. ionizer
4. collimator

3.
1aC The diameter of the X-ray beam is determined by the
1. cone size
2. lead diaphragm
3. film speed
4. kilovolt setting utilized
5. All of the above

4.
3B Fogging of a radiograph may occur due to
1. scattered secondary radiation
2. light leaks in the darkroom
3. development at temperatures in excess of 68°F
4. use of film that has passed the suggested expiration date
5. All of the above

5.
1aA Which of the following appear as radiolucent on a radiograph?
(a) carious lesions
(b) enamel
(c) marrow spaces
(d) lamina dura
1. (a), (b) and (d)
2. (a) and (c) only
3. (a), (c) and (d)
4. (c) and (d) only

6.
1aA A blurred radiograph is caused by
(a) an unsteady X-ray cone
(b) too low a kVp setting
(c) movement of the film
(d) the film being overdeveloped
1. (a) and (b)
2. (a) and (c)
3. (b) and (d)
4. (c) only
5. All of the above

7.
1aA A clear area on a radiograph is most likely caused by
1. movement of the film
2. underexposure of the film
3. cone-cutting
4. improperly fixed film

8.
1bA A treelike image on a panoramic radiograph is caused by
1. static electricity
2. light leakage into the cassette
3. cracked film
4. movement of the patient

9. Panoramic radiographs provide
1bA
   (a) less radiation exposure than a full-mouth series
   (b) good visualization of large areas of pathological conditions
   (c) good visualization of periodontal pathological conditions
   (d) a definitive survey for detection of carious lesions
   1. (a), (b) and (c)
   2. (a) and (b)
   3. (b) and (c) only
   4. (b), (c) and (d)
   5. All of the above

10. The term *paralleling technique* for exposing intraoral radiographs refers to
1aB
   1. use of a long cone
   2. the central ray being perpendicular to the film
   3. the cone opening being parallel to the film
   4. the film placed parallel to the long axis of the tooth

11. Which of the following may cause a totally clear film?
1aB
   (a) The machine was not turned on.
   (b) There was fixation before developing.
   (c) The film packet was placed in reverse.
   1. (a) and (b)
   2. (a) and (c)
   3. (b) and (c)
   4. All of the above

12. The most dangerous time to take a radiograph on a pregnant patient is during the
2A
   1. first trimester
   2. second trimester
   3. third trimester
   4. last month of pregnancy
   5. None of the above (All times are equally dangerous to the fetus.)

13. Which of the following kVp settings will produce the greatest image contrast on a radiograph?
1aC
   1. 65 kVp
   2. 80 kVp
   3. 85 kVp
   4. 90 kVp

14. A herringbone pattern appearing on a radiograph is caused by
1aB
   1. static electricity
   2. improper bending of the film during exposure
   3. the wrong side of the packet being placed toward the source of radiation
   4. the film being double exposed

15. Which of the following would most minimize the radiation dose to a patient?
1aB
   1. use of a long cone
   2. adequate filtration
   3. a lead apron over the patient's lap
   4. a film with fast emulsion speed
   5. low kilovoltage

16. Incorrect horizontal angulation of the X-ray cone will result in
1aB
   1. an elongation of the teeth on the radiograph
   2. a foreshortening of the teeth on the radiograph
   3. an overlapping of teeth on the radiograph
   4. cone-cutting of the desired image

17. Sensitivity of body tissue to radiation is related to
2A
   1. oxyhemoglobin concentration
   2. blood flow
   3. mitotic rate
   4. age of the tissue
   5. All of the above

18. **1aB** Foreshortening of a radiographic object is caused by
1. not placing the film packet parallel to the tooth
2. too much distal horizontal angulation
3. not enough vertical angulation
4. too much vertical angulation

19. **1aB** When placing a film for a periapical radiograph, the dot should be placed
1. toward the occlusal-incisal surface of the teeth
2. toward the apices of the teeth
3. toward the distal projection
4. in any area as long as the operator places it consistently

20. **1aA** Which of the following materials is radiolucent on a radiograph?
(a) porcelain
(b) acrylic
(c) silicate
(d) gutta percha
1. (a), (b) and (c)
2. (a), (b) and (d)
3. (a), (c) and (d)
4. All of the above

21. **1aC** The quantity of X-rays produced in an X-ray tube may be decreased by
1. increasing the milliamperage
2. decreasing the milliamperage
3. increasing the kilovoltage
4. decreasing the kilovoltage

22. **1aA** Bite-wing radiographs are a good diagnostic tool for detecting
(a) the extent of calculus deposits
(b) periodontitis
(c) caries
(d) gingivitis
1. (a) and (b)
2. (a) and (c)
3. (c) and (d)
4. All of the above

23. **1aB** An increase in the size of the penumbra would result in
1. an increase in the definition of the radiographic image
2. a decrease in the definition of the radiographic image
3. fogging of the radiograph
4. a decrease in density of the radiograph

24. **1aB** Magnification of the radiographic image can be minimized by
(a) using a long cone
(b) using a short cone
(c) placing the film as close to the tooth being X-rayed as possible
(d) shortening exposure time
1. (a) and (c)
2. (a), (c) and (d)
3. (b) and (c)
4. (b), (c) and (d)
5. (b) and (d)

25. **2A** When matter is irradiated by X-rays, which of the following is produced?
1. leakage radiation
2. primary radiation
3. gamma radiation
4. secondary radiation

26. **3C** Reducing the temperature of the developing solution below 68° F will result in which of the following?
1. a decrease in developing time
2. an increase in developing time
3. overdevelopment of the film
4. no effect on the developing time

27. **3B** Brownish-appearing X-ray films, stored as part of the patient's record for several months, result from
1. use of outdated film
2. improper developing and washing
3. improper fixing and washing
4. overexposure of the film

28. When positioning an intraoral film, the
3B facial side is determined by the
    1. anatomical landmarks
    2. curvature of the arch
    3. concavity of the dot
    4. convexity of the dot

29. Which of the following are landmarks
3A seen in maxillary periapical films?
    (a) maxillary sinus
    (b) zygomatic process
    (c) incisive foramen
    (d) hamular process
    1. (a), (b) and (c)
    2. (a) and (b)
    3. (b), (c) and (d)
    4. All of the above

30. The lingual foramen is a radiolucent
3A landmark usually seen
    1. between the lower premolars
    2. between the maxillary central incisors
    3. in the mandibular molar region
    4. in the mandibular anterior region

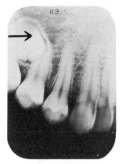

FIGURE B

32. In radiograph B, what is occurring in
5A the indicated area?
    1. A deciduous tooth is being replaced by a succedaneous tooth.
    2. A deciduous tooth has been retained.
    3. A supernumerary tooth bud has formed.
    4. A cyst has developed.

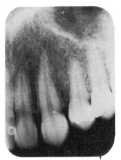

FIGURE A

31. The white line in radiograph A is
5A   1. where the film was bent
    2. the alveolar process
    3. the maxillary sinus wall
    4. the zygomatic process

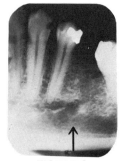

FIGURE C

33. In radiograph C, the area indicated is
5A   1. a periapical abscess
    2. the mandibular foramen
    3. the mental foramen
    4. a periodontal abscess

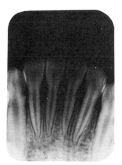

FIGURE D

34. In radiograph D, the structure most
5A adjacent to the root of tooth number
    24 is the
    1. lamina dura, which is radiopaque
    2. periodontal ligament space, which
       is radiolucent
    3. lingual foramen
    4. mandibular canal

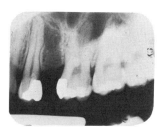

FIGURE E

35. The patient from radiograph E pre-
5A sented with throbbing pain in the
    maxillary left area. The pain was es-
    pecially pronounced when the patient
    tried to go to sleep. Ingesting hot
    liquids seemed to increase the pain.
    What was the probable source of the
    above-mentioned discomfort?
    1. the radiolucent area adjacent to
       tooth number 12
    2. the radiolucent area above tooth
       number 14

3. the vertical bone loss between
   teeth number 12 and number 14
4. the carious lesion on the distal area
   of tooth number 14

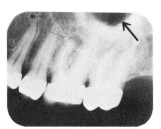

FIGURE F

36. The area indicated on radiograph F is
5A the
    1. maxillary sinus wall
    2. alveolar process
    3. zygomatic process
    4. maxillary tuberosity

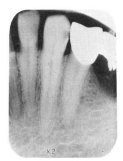

FIGURE G

37. What is the radiolucency on the distal
5A of the mandibular cuspid in radiograph
    G?
    1. a carious lesion
    2. a silicate or composite restoration
    3. an enamel defect
    4. a calcified dentinal tubule

38. A radiation detection badge is used by
2A the auxiliary taking radiographs to
1. reduce the exposure of the patient to radiation
2. protect the operator from radiation exposure
3. provide an estimate of the radiation absorbed by the operator
4. All of the above

39. Film exposed to light during the devel-
3B opment process will be
1. light
2. black
3. clear
4. blurred

40. Receiving small amounts of radiation
2A over an extended period
1. decreases the relative radiosensitivity of different cells
2. results in biological damage
3. allows time for tissue repair
4. affects fertility
5. Both (2) and (3) above

41. If your patient has just had a full mouth
2A radiographic survey, when should another be taken?
1. in 6 months
2. yearly
3. every 2 years
4. every 5 years
5. when indicated

42. The MPD (maximum permissible
2A dose) of radiation is
1. 0.1 rem/year
2. 0.5 rem/year
3. 1.0 rem/year
4. 5.0 rem/year

43. The thin, regular, radiopaque line sur-
5A rounding the periodontal membrane space is the
1. alveolar bone proper
2. periodontal ligament
3. cellular cementum
4. lamina dura

44. The characteristics of periodontal dis-
5A ease that can be determined radiographically are
   (a) horizontal bone loss
   (b) periodontal abscess formation
   (c) thickening of the periodontal ligament
   (d) gingival recession
1. (a) and (b)
2. (a), (b) and (c)
3. (a), (b) and (d)
4. (a) and (c)
5. All of the above

45. Injury to a tooth by radiation during its
5A development can result in
1. hypercementosis
2. radiation caries
3. amelogenesis imperfecta
4. partial odontia
5. None of the above

46. Reticulation of dental radiographs indi-
3B cates that
1. there was inadequate time provided in the developing solution
2. there was inadequate fixation time
3. there were sudden temperature changes during fixation
4. the film was improperly exposed

47.   Discoloration of radiographs may be
3B   due to
or   (a)   incomplete processing
3C   (b)   incomplete rinsing
         (c)   storage of the film in an area
               that is too warm
         (d)   storage of the film near con-
               taminating chemicals
      1.   (a) and (b)
      2.   (a), (b) and (c)
      3.   (b) and (d)
      4.   All of the above

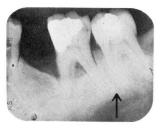

FIGURE H

48.   The area indicated by the arrow in
5A   radiograph H represents
      1.   a defect caused by a tooth extrac-
           tion
      2.   horizontal bone loss due to peri-
           odontal disease
      3.   a periodontal abscess
      4.   vertical bone loss due to periodon-
           tal disease

Chapter 3

Providing Other Diagnostic Aids

With recent expansion in the scope of duties of the dental hygienist, there are other diagnostic aids that must be understood in order for the hygienist to effectively carry out his or her duties in the dental practice. These include various diagnostic tests to be administered and preparation of study casts. On the National Board Dental Hygiene Examination there are 32 questions devoted to this general category. These are classified in the chart so that you can see the emphasis placed on certain areas.

Function	Questions and Categories
1. Obtaining medical and dental health histories (tests, vital signs, emotional status, etc.)	18 questions 16-A; 2-B
2. Preparing study casts a. taking impressions b. pour, trim and mount	9 questions 3-A; 2-B; 2-C 1-A; 1-B
3. Clinical testing (thermal, vitalometer, percussion, transillumination, caries activity, cytologic smear, etc.)	5 questions 3-A; 2-B

A=background information
B=methodology
C=armamentarium

Recommended References

Castano, F. A., and Alden, B. A. *Handbook of clinical dental auxiliary practice*. Philadelphia: Lippincott, 1980.

Physicians Desk Reference, 1982.

Wilkins, E. *Clinical practice of the dental hygienist*. Philadelphia: Lea & Febiger, 1976.

Woodall, I. et al. *Comprehensive dental hygiene care*. St. Louis: C. V. Mosby, 1980.

Questions

1.   The artery in the arm used to obtain a
1A   blood pressure reading is the
     1.   brachial artery
     2.   radial artery
     3.   carotid artery
     4.   ulnar artery

2.   The cuff pressure should continue to
1B   be released slowly for about __mm
     after the last sound is heard, to asssure
     cessation of all sounds.
     1.   10
     2.   20
     3.   30
     4.   40

3.   When applying the blood pressure
1B   cuff, the patient's arm should be
          (a)   elevated
          (b)   at or below the level of the
                heart
          (c)   on the patient's lap
          (d)   on a level surface
     1.   (a) and (c)
     2.   (a) and (d)
     3.   (b) and (d)
     4.   (b) only

4.   When deflating the cuff to obtain the
1B   blood pressure reading, the air lock
     should be released about __mm per
     second, so that the dial or mercury
     drops gradually.
     1.   2–3
     2.   3–5
     3.   5–7
     4.   7–9

5.   Which of the following statements de-
1B   scribes accurate blood pressure cuff
     placement on the patient's arm? The
     lower edge of the cuff
     1.   is 2 inches above the antecubital
          fossa.
     2.   is 1 inch above the antecubital
          fossa.
     3.   covers the antecubital fossa.
     4.   is 1 inch below the antecubital
          fossa.

6.   The current accepted approach recog-
1B   nized by the American Heart Associa-
     tion to prophylactic antibiotic therapy
     is to give
          (a)   2.0 gm of penicillin to the pa-
                tient orally 30 minutes to 1
                hour prior to the procedure
                and then 500 mg orally every 6
                hours for 8 doses
          (b)   500 mg of penicillin to the pa-
                tient four times a day, 2 days
                prior to the dental procedure
                and for 2 days following the
                procedure
          (c)   1.0 gm of erythromycin orally
                1½–2 hours prior to the proce-
                dure and then 500 mg orally
                every 6 hours for 8 doses
     1.   (a) and (b)
     2.   (a) and (c)
     3.   (b) and (c)
     4.   All of the above

7. Antibiotic coverage is usually given
1A prior to any dental treatment that is
undertaken on a patient with a positive
history of
    (a) hepatitis
    (b) diabetes
    (c) congenital heart disease
    (d) rheumatic fever
  1. (a), (b) and (d)
  2. (a), (c) and (d)
  3. (b) and (c)
  4. (c) and (d)
  5. All of the above

8. A patient who has epilepsy is often
1A treated with the anticonvulsant drug
  1. phenobarbital
  2. diphenylhydantoin
  3. epinephrine
  4. chlordiazepoxide
  5. None of the above

9. Retarded wound healing can be ex-
1A pected in a patient suffering from
  1. epilepsy
  2. angina pectoris
  3. diabetes
  4. tuberculosis

10. The normal pulse rate of an adult is
1A 1. 40–50 beats per minute
  2. 60–80 beats per minute
  3. 90–110 beats per minute
  4. 115–125 beats per minute

11. If a 2-year-old child has an infection for
1A which antibiotic therapy is required,
the least desirable drug to use is
  1. ampicillin
  2. penicillin
  3. tetracycline
  4. erythromycin

12. The most common cause of a high met-
1A abolic rate is
  1. hyperthyroidism
  2. hormonal imbalance
  3. hypothyroidism
  4. hyperparathyroidism

13. When using a sphygmomanometer,
1B systolic pressure is indicated by the
  1. first audible sound
  2. last audible sound
  3. fading of the sound
  4. pulsation of the mercury column

14. The use of a transillumination device
3A on anterior teeth is useful in detection
of
    (a) pulpal inflammation
    (b) interproximal caries
    (c) supporting bone levels
    (d) calculus deposits
  1. (a) and (b)
  2. (a), (b) and (d)
  3. (b) and (c)
  4. (b) and (d)
  5. All of the above

15. Drugs are listed in the *PDR (Physi-*
1A *cians Desk Reference)*
    (a) by manufacturer's name
    (b) by brand name
    (c) alphabetically
    (d) by generic name
  1. (a), (b) and (c)
  2. (b), (c) and (d)
  3. (c) and (d) only
  4. All of the above

16. The setting of alginate impression ma-
2A terial is the result of
  1. gelation
  2. syneresis
  3. polymerization
  4. hydrocolloidization

17. An alginate impression would distort
2A least if stored briefly in which of the
following ways?
 1. a bowl of water
 2. moist towels
 3. an isotonic saline solution
 4. a refrigerator

18. The primary purpose for using a vibra-
2bA tor when pouring alginate impressions
in dental stone or plaster is to
 1. eliminate distortion
 2. eliminate trapped air
 3. increase the setting time
 4. slow down the setting time

19. Decreasing the water temperature
2aA when mixing alginate impression material
 1. makes it a firmer impression medium
 2. increases the setting time
 3. decreases the setting time
 4. increases the likeliness of distortion

20. Involuntary movements of the facial
1A muscles and the tongue may be associated with a condition called
 1. tic douloureaux
 2. Bell's palsy
 3. tardive dyskinesia
 4. dysphasia

21. Consultation with the patient's physi-
1A cian because of danger of hemorrhag-
ing if a prophylaxis is performed would
be indicated if the medical history
showed that the patient was taking the
drug
 (a) thrombin
 (b) Coumadin
 (c) heparin
 (d) fibrin
 1. (a) and (b)
 2. (a) and (c)
 3. (b) and (c)
 4. (b) and (d)
 5. All of the above

22. Which of the following are necessary in
3B the proper procedure of oral exfoliative
cytology testing?
 (a) The lesion should be scraped
 with a tongue blade to pick up
 cells.
 (b) The tongue blade should be
 wiped back and forth across a
 slide several times.
 (c) The exfoliated cells should be
 smeared on two slides.
 (d) The slide should be air dried
 and then placed in a fixative.
 1. (a), (b) and (c)
 2. (a) and (b) only
 3. (a) and (c) only
 4. All of the above

23. If a patient's medical history indicated
1A that he or she was using the drug glyc-
eryl trinitrate (nitroglycerin), this
would indicate that the patient was being treated for
 1. epilepsy
 2. neurosis
 3. congenital heart disease
 4. angina pectoris
 5. None of the above

24. If the dental hygienist determined that
1A the patient was taking the above-
mentioned drug, the treatment plan
 1. would prohibit a prophylaxis procedure for this patient
 2. would require prophylactic antibiotic coverage for this patient
 3. would indicate that the drug
 should be placed on the bracket
 table for easy access
 4. need not be altered for the procedures of the prophylaxis appointment

25.
1A

Clumping of cells causing bulging in the papilla is indicative that the patient suffers from which of the following conditions?
1. coronary thrombosis
2. leukemia
3. hemophilia
4. diabetes

26.
1A

A 68-year-old woman presents for a long overdue recall appointment. An update of the medical and dental histories indicates that she has had a heart condition, which necessitated placement of a pacemaker. Because of her infirmity, she has neglected all oral hygiene and has extensive deposits of calculus and plaque with gingival inflammation. The treatment plan of choice would be
1. at the first appointment, to instruct the patient in home care only
2. to use an ultrasonic scaling device to begin debridement of her mouth and provide her relief quickly
3. to begin scaling with hand instruménts and schedule several appointments for dental hygiene therapy
4. to schedule another appointment following antibiotic coverage

27.
1A

A patient presents for an initial appointment. The dental hygienist notices a characteristic fruity odor (acetone) to the breath. The patient probably suffers from
1. epilepsy
2. diabetes
3. tuberculosis
4. coronary heart disease

28.
1A

Further oral inspection of this patient may be expected to reveal
(a) gingival hyperplasia
(b) dry mucosa
(c) excessive plaque and calculus deposits
(d) exaggerated inflammatory response to the presence of local irritants
1. (a), (b) and (c)
2. (b), (c) and (d)
3. (b) and (d) only
4. All of the above

29.
1B

Appointment planning for this patient should include
(a) more frequent recall appointments
(b) appointments 1½ hours after mealtime
(c) a series of appointments if extensive instrumentation is required
(d) nutritional counseling if instrumentation causes difficulty in eating solid foods
1. (a) and (b)
2. (b) and (c)
3. (c) and (d)
4. All of the above

30. If soft tissue curettage is required on
1B this patient, which of the following
    should be done?
    (a) The patient should be given
        antibiotics to aid in healing
    (b) If an anesthetic is needed for
        the procedure, one without
        epinephrine should be used
    (c) appropriate rinses should be
        utilized to make the patient
        more comfortable
    (d) the hygienist should take nec-
        essary precautions for a poten-
        tial emergency
    1. (a), (b) and (d)
    2. (a), (c) and (d)
    3. (b), (c) and (d)
    4. All of the above

31. Which of the following clinical obser-
3A vations would most likely indicate a
    need to perform a pulp vitality test?
    1. apical radiographic opacity
    2. a large amalgam restoration
    3. discoloration of a tooth
    4. increased occlusal wear

32. Which of the following sources would
3A you include in assessing tooth vital-
or ity?
3B   (a) medical history
        (b) dental history
        (c) clinical examination
        (d) radiographs
        (e) hot and cold testing
    1. (a), (b) and (d)
    2. (a), (c) and (e)
    3. (b), (c) and (d)
    4. (b), (d) and (e)
    5. All of the above

33. Mr. Jones presents with discomfort in
3B tooth number 3. He describes it as an
    intermittent throbbing pain. Your oral
    inspection shows tooth number 3 with
    cervical abrasion and a Class V amal-
    gam restoration. In addition, you ob-
    serve an M/O inlay with a composite
    restoration at its distal border.
    Dr. Smith recommends that a pulp vi-
    tality test be performed. Which of the
    following areas should be tested?
    1. area of cervical abrasion
    2. occlusal surface
    3. all of the teeth on the same arch
    4. middle one-third of each cusp on
       tooth number 3

34. A Snyder's test suggesting marked car-
3A ies susceptibility indicates that the pa-
    tient
    1. is in need of immediate restorative
       treatment
    2. should be instructed to use dental
       floss
    3. must be put on a sucrose-free
       diet
    4. None of the above

35. After 72 hours of incubating, a very low
3A pH value (i.e., high acidity) in the Sny-
or der test agar suggests
3B 1. no caries susceptibility
    2. slight caries susceptibility
    3. moderate caries susceptibility
    4. very great caries susceptibility

Chapter 4

Performing Prophylaxis

The dental hygienist is constantly involved with *prophylactic procedures* in the dental operatory. These procedures entail such methods and techniques as scaling and root planing, soft tissue curettage, and polishing. Because so much of a routine appointment involves prophylaxis, various aspects are treated on the National Board Examination, including pertinent background information and methodology. In addition, there are specific instruments in the armamentarium with which you must be thoroughly familiar. These aspects are classified in the chart and encompass 43 questions.

Function	Questions and Categories
1. Scaling and root planing	30 questions 12-**A**; 12-**B**; 6-**C**
2. Soft tissue curettage	9 questions 6-**A**; 3-**B**
3. Polishing (coronal surfaces and appliances)	4 questions 1-**A**; 2-**B**; 1-**C**

A=background information
B=methodology
C=armamentarium

Recommended References

Parr, R., et al. *Subgingival scaling and root planning*. San Francisco: University of Calif., 1976.

Pattison, G., and Pattison, A. *Periodontal instrumentation*. Reston, Va.: Reston Publishing, 1979.

Wilkins, E. *Clinical practice of the dental hygienist*. Philadelphia: Lea & Febiger, 1983.

Woodall, I., et al. *Comprehensive dental hygiene care*. St. Louis: C. V. Mosby, 1980.

Questions

1. Definitive soft tissue curettage is con-
2A traindicated in the presence of
    1. suprabony pockets
    2. shallow pockets of 4–6 mm
    3. deep infrabony pockets
    4. soft, spongy, edematous tissue

2. The objectives of root planing are to
1A   (a) eliminate affected cementum
    (b) remove calculus embedded in the cementum
    (c) remove large deposits of calculus
    (d) smoothe the root surface
    1. (a), (b) and (c)
    2. (a), (b) and (d)
    3. (a), (c) and (d)
    4. (b), (c) and (d)
    5. All of the above

3. Which of the following instruments
1C should be used in the final evaluation of the root surface?
    1. universal curette
    2. sickle
    3. explorer
    4. gracey curette

4. In performing definitive soft tissue cu-
2B rettage, the angle of the blade against the tissue should be
    1. less than 45°
    2. 45–90°
    3. 90–110°
    4. greater than 110°

5. In polishing, the following technique
3B should be used:
    1. The rubber cup should reach the bottom of the sulcus.
    2. The cup should slip slightly subgingivally.
    3. Brushes should be used for the gingival third.
    4. Apply high speed and light pressure.

6. Which of the following instruments
1C can be used to detect furcation involvement?
    (a) periodontal probe
    (b) Nabers probe
    (c) curette
    (d) file
    1. (a), (b) and (c)
    2. (a), (c) and (d)
    3. (b), (c) and (d)
    4. All of the above

7. The objective of definitive soft tissue
2A curettage is the removal of
    (a) diseased connective tissue
    (b) diseased cementum
    (c) sulcular epithelium
    (d) granulomatous tissue
    1. (a), (b) and (c)
    2. (a), (c) and (d)
    3. (b), (c) and (d)
    4. (b) and (c)

8. Ultrasonic instruments are advanta-
1A geous for the following reasons:
    (a) They are fast in the removal of large deposits.
    (b) They require less effort on the part of the operator in the removal of stain and supragingival deposits.
    (c) They cause less trauma and postoperative pain.
    (d) A light stroke can be used, which increases tactile sensitivity.
    1. (a), (b) and (c)
    2. (a), (c) and (d)
    3. (b), (c) and (d)
    4. All of the above

9. The following is true of the ultrasonic
1B scaler. It
    1. is capable of complete, definitive root planing.
    2. eliminates the need for hand instrumentation
    3. uses a slow, meticulous stroke
    4. is ideal for patients with ANUG

10. The single best criterion for evaluating
1A the success of root planing two weeks
     posttreatment is
     1. lack of accumulation of supra- and
        submarginal plaque
     2. shrinkage of the pocket depth
     3. no evidence of sulcular bleeding
        upon probing
     4. a smooth and glasslike appearance
        of the root

11. Which of the following statements de-
1B scribe the differences between a work-
     ing (scaling) stroke and a root planing
     stroke?
     (a) The blade of the working
         stroke is 45–90° to the tooth;
         the root planing stroke uses a
         45–60° blade angle.
     (b) The working stroke uses heavy
         pressure; the root planing
         stroke uses light pressure.
     (c) The working stroke uses a long
         stroke; the root planing stroke
         uses a short stroke.
     (d) The working stroke is used on
         crowns and large deposits; the
         planing stroke is used on ce-
         mentum and/or dentin.
     1. (a), (b) and (c)
     2. (a), (b) and (d)
     3. (a), (c) and (d)
     4. (b), (c) and (d)
     5. None of the above

12. Which of the following statements de-
1A scribe the difference between a gracey
     curette and a universal curette?
     (a) The universal curette is used
         for scaling only; the gracey is
         used for root planing only.
     (b) The gracey has one working
         cutting blade on each end; the
         universal has two working
         blades on each end.
     (c) The gracey curette is area spe-
         cific; the universal is designed
         for work on all areas.
     (d) The gracey blade is angled 60-
         70° to the shank; the universal
         is angled at 90° to the shank.
     1. (a), (b) and (c)
     2. (a), (c) and (d)
     3. (b), (c) and (d)
     4. (a), (b) and (d)
     5. All of the above

13. Following definitive soft tissue curet-
2A tage, the most common healing re-
     sponse is
     1. reduction of pocket depth by
        shrinkage of edematous tissue
     2. regeneration of attachement
     3. regeneration of Sharpey's fibers
     4. formation of a long junctional epi-
        thelium

14. Dull instruments contribute to
1C
    (a) burnished calculus
    (b) heavy-handedness
    (c) longer operating time
    (d) the likelihood of slippage and trauma
  1. (a), (b) and (c)
  2. (a), (c) and (d)
  3. (b), (c) and (d)
  4. (a), (b) and (d)
  5. All of the above

15. The amount of pressure used in engine
3B polishing is
3C
  1. light and intermittent
  2. light and constant
  3. heavier on anterior than posterior teeth
  4. heavier on posterior than anterior teeth

16. Which of the following instruments is
1C recommended for removal of supragingival calculus and subgingival calculus that is 1–2 mm thick?
  1. hoe
  2. file
  3. sickle
  4. curette

17. The ultrasonic scaler has a positive in-
1A fluence on tissue response. This is most likely due to
    (a) the flushing action of the water lavage on debris
    (b) the coagulation of the necrotic soft tissue
    (c) lack of trauma from cutting, since the instrument is not sharp
    (d) lack of trauma from pressure, since only light pressure is required
  1. (a), (b) and (c)
  2. (a), (c) and (d)
  3. (b), (c) and (d)
  4. All of the above
  5. None of the above

18. The criterion for determining if teeth
3A need to be polished is the amount of
  1. plaque present
  2. caries present
  3. endogenous stain
  4. extrinsic stain

19. Burnished calculus is most likely the
1B result of
  1. the inability of the operator to maintain sufficient lateral pressure
  2. an insufficient number of exploratory strokes
  3. using too sharp an instrument
  4. using a hoe instead of a curette

1B Test items 20 through 23 refer to the diagrams below.

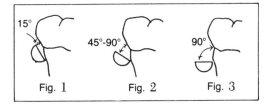

Fig. 1   Fig. 2   Fig. 3

Which of the diagrams above represents the correct angulation for the following?

20. _____ working stroke

21. _____ exploring stroke

22. _____ planing stroke

23. _____ soft tissue curettage

24. Many instruments can be used in the
1C removal of deposits from teeth. Which
one of the following has been shown to
produce the smoothest root surface
while inflicting the *least* amount of
damage?
    1. file
    2. sickle
    3. hoe
    4. curette

25. Fourteen days after definitive soft tis-
2A sue curettage, which of the following
would you expect?
    (a) no evidence of bleeding upon
        probing
    (b) clinically normal pink color
    (c) no edema
    (d) histologically complete epithe-
        lialization
    1. (a), (b) and (c)
    2. (a) and (d)
    3. (b) and (c)
    4. (a), (b) and (d)
    5. All of the above

26. A patient exhibits large amounts of
1A bacterial plaque (using the 2 dye stain,
the plaque turns blue) on the gingival third, but there is no calculus, no
pocket formation, no bleeding upon
probing, and no other clinical signs of
inflammation. The most probable
cause for the patient's state of health is
that the patient must
    1. normally brush well but did not do
       so on this day
    2. have large amounts of Vitamin C
       in his or her diet
    3. have a high level of resistance to
       the plaque
    4. have routine prophylaxis at least
       once every four months

27. A patient exhibits involved periodontal
1A disease in which four to five appointments are needed for root planing and
curettage. A successful result will be
most likely if the following procedures
and concepts are incorporated into the
appointments:
    (a) The tissue previously instru-
        mented is re-evaluated at the
        next appointment.
    (b) The patient is involved in the
        evaluation process.
    (c) Patient education is reinforced
        at each appointment.
    (d) The patient is made to realize
        that regular 6-month cleanings
        are essential.
    1. (a), (b) and (c)
    2. (a), (c) and (d)
    3. (b), (c) and (d)
    4. (a), (b) and (d)
    5. All of the above

28. After removal of large deposits of cal-
1B culus from the roots, final smoothing
and planing of the roots must be done
because
    (a) the working stroke often leaves
        grooves or ridges
    (b) submarginal calculus is at-
        tached *in* the cementum rather
        than *on* it
    (c) submarginal calculus is at-
        tached by a primary cuticle,
        which must be removed
    (d) altered cementum must be re-
        moved and planed to allow
        healing
    1. (a), (b) and (c)
    2. (a), (b) and (d)
    3. (b), (c) and (d)
    4. All of the above
    5. None of the above

29. **2A** The following are acceptable proce-dures:
   (a) performing root planing and definitive soft tissue curettage at the same appointment
   (b) performing root planing first, and definitive soft tissue curet-tage at a later appointment
   (c) performing soft tissue curet-tage first, and root planing at a later appointment
   (d) performing scaling, root plan-ing, and plaque control, then evaluating the need for defini-tive curettage
   1. (a), (b) and (c)
   2. (a), (b) and (d)
   3. (a), (c) and (d)
   4. (b), (c) and (d)
   5. All of the above

30. **1B** A finishing file is best sharpened by a
   (a) flat Arkansas stone
   (b) flat ruby stone
   (c) moonstone
   (d) Neivert whitler
   1. (a), (b) and (c)
   2. (a), (c) and (d)
   3. (b), (c) and (d)
   4. All of the above
   5. None of the above

31. **1C** The contra-angled sickle is designed primarily for use on the
   1. interproximal of anterior teeth
   2. interproximal of posterior teeth
   3. lingual and buccal surfaces
   4. deep interproximal pockets of pos-terior teeth

32. **2A** Lack of success in the outcome of de-finitive soft tissue curettage may be due to
   (a) regrowth of bacterial plaque
   (b) rapid downgrowth of new epi-thelium
   (c) incomplete removal of junc-tional and pocket epithelium
   (d) incomplete removal of calculus and/or altered cementum
   1. (a), (b) and (c)
   2. (a), (c) and (d)
   3. (a), (b) and (d)
   4. (b), (c) and (d)
   5. All of the above

33. **1B** A gracey instrument is correctly adapted when the
   1. upper shank is parallel to the long axis of the tooth
   2. handle is parallel to the long axis of the tooth
   3. angle of the blade to the tooth is 40°
   4. lower shank is parallel with the tooth surface being scaled

34. **1A** The *primary* reason for removing cal-culus from root surfaces is because it
   1. acts as a mechanical irritant against the soft tissue
   2. harbors plaque organisms
   3. pushes down against the junc-tional epithelium
   4. alters the cementum

35. Whether enamel or cementum is re-
3A moved during polishing depends on
    1. the type of abrasive used
    2. the use of brushes
    3. how much pressure is used
    4. how dry the teeth are kept

36. The significance of bleeding upon
1A probing relates to the
    (a) depth of the periodontal pock-
        et
    (b) ulcerated epithelial lining
    (c) toxic by-products that have
        reached the deeper parts of the
        periodontium
    (d) patient not having flossed
    1. (a) and (b)
    2. (a) and (d)
    3. (b) and (c)
    4. (c) and (d)
    5. None of the above

37. A sterile sharpening stone should be
1C part of a hygienist's working armamen-
    tarium *because* instruments are dulled
    during instrumentation.
    1. Both statement and reason are
       correct and related.
    2. Both statement and reason are
       correct but *not* related.
    3. The statement is correct, but the
       reason is not.
    4. The statement is not correct, but
       the reason is accurate.
    5. Neither the statement nor the rea-
       son is correct.

38. In root planing, a smoother surface is
1B more likely to result if which of the fol-
    lowing procedures is employed?
    1. a wide variety of overlapping
       strokes
    2. vertical strokes
    3. horizontal strokes
    4. oblique strokes

39. The primary cause of periodontal dis-
1A ease is
    1. occlusal trauma
    2. calculus formation
    3. bacterial plaque
    4. improper brushing

40. In soft tissue curettage on the lingual
2B and facial, the blade should be directed
    toward the tissue and the stroke should
    be
    1. short and vertical, with heavy
       pressure
    2. long and oblique, with moderate
       pressure
    3. short and horizontal, with moder-
       ate pressure
    4. long and horizontal, with moder-
       ate pressure

41. Gingival inflammation is primarily
1A caused by
    1. bacterial invasion
    2. calculus formation
    3. occlusal trauma
    4. toxic bacterial by-products

42. Definitive curettage is performed with a
2B
  1. Hirschfield file
  2. hoe
  3. Black's gold knife
  4. universal curette

43. Ultrasonic scalers are ideally suited for
1A patients with cardiac pacemakers *because* they utilize blunt tips.
  1. Both statement and reason are correct and related.
  2. Neither the statement nor the reason is related.
  3. Both statement and reason are correct but *not* related.
  4. The statement is correct, but the reason is not.
  5. None of the above

44. When sharpening a curette, the angle
1B between the face of the blade and the stone is
  1. 70–80°
  2. 90°
  3. 100–110°
  4. 110–120°

Chapter 5

Applying Topical Agents

Frequently, caries prevention calls for the *application of topical agents*. Topical anesthetics and tooth desensitization also require expert knowledge in the application of various topical agents. On the National Board Examination there are 17 questions pertaining to this subject area as outlined in the chart on this page.

Function	Questions and Categories
1. Caries preventive	11 questions 7-**A**; 3-**B**; 1-**C**
2. Anesthetic	3 questions 2-**A**; 1-**B**
3. Tooth desensitizing	3 questions 2-**A**; 1-**B**

A=background information
B=methodology
C=armamentarium

Recommended References

American Dental Association. *Accepted dental therapeutics*. Chicago: 1982.

Pattison, G., and Pattison, A. *Periodontal instrumentation: a clinical manual*. Reston, Va.: Reston Publishing, 1979.

Wilkins, E. *Clinical practice of the dental hygienist*. Philadelphia: Lea & Febiger, 1983.

Woodall, I., et al. *Comprehensive dental hygiene care*. St. Louis: C. V. Mosby, 1980.

Questions

1. Which of the following would contrain-
1B dicate the application of pit and fissure
sealants?
    (a)   many proximal lesions
    (b)   deep narrow pits
    (c)   teeth that have been caries-
         free for four or more years
    (d)   well-coalesced pits
    1. (a), (b) and (c)
    2. (a), (b) and (d)
    3. (a), (c) and (d)
    4. (b), (c) and (d)
    5. None of the above

2. Ultraviolet light is often used in which
1C of the following techniques?
    1. placement of periodontal packs
    2. placement of amalgams
    3. pit and fissure sealants
    4. placement of ZOE restorations

3. Which of the following is the least de-
2A sirable form of topical anesthetic?
    1. gel
    2. spray
    3. liquid
    4. ointment

4. Methods for treating hypersensitivity
3B are aimed at the following mecha-
nisms:
    (a)   denaturing the peripheral ends
         of Tomes' fibers in dentin
    (b)   depositing an insoluble mate-
         rial at the ends of tubules
    (c)   stimulating dentin formation
    (d)   using antibiotics for inflamma-
         tion in the gingiva
    1. (a), (b) and (c)
    2. (a), (c) and (d)
    3. (b), (c) and (d)
    4. All of the above
    5. None of the above

5. Which of the following statements are
1A true of stannous fluoride as a topical
agent?
    (a)   An 8% solution should be used
         twice a year.
    (b)   A fresh solution must be mixed
         each time.
    (c)   It stains radiographs.
    (d)   It may cause gingival irrita-
         tions.
    (e)   It stains hypocalcified enamel
         and silicate restorations.
    1. (a), (b), (c) and (d)
    2. (a), (b), (d) and (e)
    3. (b), (c), (d) and (e)
    4. All of the above
    5. None of the above

6. The addition of fluoride to a prophy-
1B laxis paste cannot reliably be said to
produce protection from decay *because* fluoride is often deactivated by
the abrasive or other paste ingredients.
    1. The statement is true; the reason
       is false.
    2. Both statement and reason are
       true, but not related.
    3. Both statement and reason are
       true and related.
    4. The statement is false, but the rea-
       son is true.
    5. Neither the statement nor the rea-
       son is true.

7. It has been shown that it is *not* always
1B necessary to polish teeth prior to giving a fluoride treatment *because* fluoride is able to penetrate through
plaque and acquired pellicle.
    1. Both statement and reason are
       correct, but not related.
    2. Both statement and reason are
       correct and related.
    3. The statement is correct; the rea-
       son is not.
    4. Neither the statement nor the rea-
       son is correct.

8. For home use, limitation on each pre-
1A scription should be no more than
   1. 360 mg of stannous fluoride
   2. 220 mg of sodium fluoride
   3. 160 mg of acidulated phosphate fluoride
   4. 264 mg of sodium fluoride

9. The following ingredient(s), in some
3A form, has (have) been reported to have some degree of success in the treatment of hypersensitivity:
   1. fluoride
   2. strontium chloride
   3. formaldehyde
   4. sodium monofluorophosphate
   5. All of the above

10. Topical applications of fluoride can
1A produce the following:
   (a) calcium fluoride
   (b) fluorapatite
   (c) an antibacterial effect on plaque
   (d) remineralization
   1. (a), (b) and (c)
   2. (a), (c) and (d)
   3. (b), (c) and (d)
   4. All of the above
   5. None of the above

11. Which of the following considerations
1B is the most important during a fluoride application? The teeth must be
   1. polished thoroughly before the application
   2. dried thoroughly before the application
   3. kept constantly wet with the fluoride
   4. flossed during the application

12. The following is true of iontophoresis:
3B   1. The pulp tester is used for the electric charge.
   2. Sodium chloride is used in this technique.
   3. It encourages negative ions to penetrate the tooth surface.
   4. It is safe to use on people with pacemakers.

13. Which of the following statements are
2A true of topical anesthetics?
   (a) There is a higher concentration of anesthetic agents as compared to local anesthesia.
   (b) They are readily absorbed through keratinized epithelium.
   (c) They are easily swallowed and can create a numb throat.
   (d) They act on terminal nerve endings.
   1. (a), (b) and (c)
   2. (a), (c) and (d)
   3. (b), (c) and (d)
   4. All of the above
   5. None of the above

14. After polishing, it is important to give a
1B fluoride rinse or topical treatment *because* the outermost layers of enamel, which are the richest in fluoride concentration, have been removed.
   1. The statement is correct; the reason is false.
   2. Both statement and reason are correct, but not related.
   3. Both statement and reason are correct and related.
   4. The statement is false, but the reason is true.

15. Which of the following is recommend-
1A ed for weekly home rinses?
    1. 0.05% neutral sodium fluoride
    2. 0.2% neutral sodium fluoride
    3. 0.02% neutral sodium fluoride
    4. 1.23% neutral stannous fluoride

16. Dental fluorosis is caused by an excess
1A of fluoride
    1. applied topically
    2. ingested prenatally (mother to fe-
       tus)
    3. during the pre-eruptive, but post-
       calcification period
    4. during the calcification period

17. Which of the following statements are
3A true in the treatment of hypersensitiv-
    ity?
    (a) The exact mechanism of pain
        transmission is not known.
    (b) There are no accepted prod-
        ucts or recognized treatments.
    (c) Fluorides in several forms
        have been effective.
    (d) The area closest to the DEJ
        (dentinoenamel junction) ap-
        pears to be the most sensi-
        tive.
    1. (a), (b) and (c)
    2. (a), (c) and (d)
    3. (b), (c) and (d)
    4. All of the above
    5. None of the above

18. Which of the following is contraindi-
1B cated before the application of a pit and
    fissure sealant?
    (a) polishing with pumice and
        water
    (b) polishing with a fluoride paste
    (c) fluoride treatment
    (d) fluoride rinse
    1. (a), (b) and (c)
    2. (a), (b) and (d)
    3. (a), (c) and (d)
    4. (b), (c) and (d)
    5. None of the above

19. Acidulated phosphate gels and solu-
1A tions have the following content:
    1. 1.23% of fluoride and a pH of 5.7
    2. 1% fluoride and a pH of 4.2
    3. 1.23% fluoride and a pH of 3.5
    4. 0.2% fluoride and a pH of 7.2

20. The proper procedure in applying a
2B topical anesthetic is to
    (a) dry the tissue and apply it lib-
        erally to one quadrant with a
        cotton swab
    (b) dry the tissue and allow it to
        flow interproximally or subgin-
        givally
    (c) apply it to a limited area
    (d) apply a limited amount
    1. (a), (b) and (c)
    2. (a), (c) and (d)
    3. (b), (c) and (d)
    4. All of the above
    5. None of the above

21. The unit crystal that is primarily af-
1A fected by fluoride in the prevention of
    decay is
    1. calcium
    2. phosphorus
    3. hydroxyapatite
    4. calcium phosphate

22. The highest concentration of dental
1A fluoride is found in the
    1. outer parts of the enamel
    2. inner parts of the enamel
    3. dentin
    4. cementum

Chapter 6

Providing Individual Oral Health Instruction

As a health care provider, one of the most important roles that the dental hygienist assumes is that of educator. As a health care educator and provider, you may be called upon to identify a need for counseling in oral health, as well as either planning and/or providing instruction in oral hygiene. You will also need to know how to evaluate and follow up on any instruction that you may provide.

Encompassed in the broad topic of *oral health instruction* are 56 questions on the National Board Examination. Included in this section are questions on such items as nutrition and plaque control. Emphasis on the various items is detailed in the chart.

Function	Questions and Categories
1. Identifying needs for counseling	24 questions 19-**A**; 5-**B**
2. Planning instruction	13 questions - **A**
3. Providing instruction	10 questions 8-**B**; 2-**C**
4. Evaluating instruction	9 questions 4-**A**; 5-**B**

A-background information
B-methodology
C-armamentarium

Recommended References

American Academy of Pedodontics. *Changing perspectives in nutrition and caries research*. New York: Medcom, 1979.

American Dental Hygienists Association. *Nutrition, diet and dental health: concepts and methods*. (Self-study Course.) 1981.

Nizel, *Nutrition in preventive dentistry*. Philadelphia: W. B. Saunders, 1981.

Pipe, et al. *Developing a plaque control program*. Berkeley: Praxis Publishing, 1972.

Randolph, P. M., and Dennison, I. *Diet, nutrition and dentistry*. St. Louis: C. V. Mosby, 1981.

Wilkins, *Clinical practice of the dental hygienist*. Philadelphia: Lea & Febiger, 1976.

Williams, S. R. *Essentials of nutrition and diet therapy*. St. Louis: C. V. Mosby, 1982.

Woodall, I. et al. *Comprehensive dental hygiene care*. St. Louis: C. V. Mosby, 1980.

Questions

1.
1A If a patient presents for examination with moderate amounts of plaque but with no change in gingival contour or texture and no bleeding upon probing, which of the following statements would characterize the patient? The patient
   1. does not use a disclosing solution or tablets
   2. is using the wrong toothbrushing technique
   3. brushes regularly but does not floss
   4. has not brushed and flossed within the last 24-hour period

2.
3B If, upon the use of a disclosing agent, it is noted that the patient has plaque accumulation only at the cervical one-third of the teeth, the toothbrushing method of choice would be
   1. roll
   2. Fone's
   3. Bass
   4. Modified Stillman's

3.
2A Digestion begins in the mouth for which of the following?
   1. starch
   2. protein
   3. lipids
   4. glucose

4.
2A Which of the following carbohydrates influences caries development?
   (a) fructose
   (b) lactose
   (c) sucrose
   (d) glucose
   1. (a) and (b)
   2. (b) and (c)
   3. (c) and (d)
   4. All of the above

5.
1A Which of the following nutrients has an important role in wound healing?
   (a) vitamin B
   (b) protein
   (c) folic acid
   (d) vitamin C
   1. (a) and (b)
   2. (b) and (c)
   3. (b) and (d)
   4. All of the above

6.
4B The best way to evaluate the ability of your patient in mastering oral physio-therapy techniques would be to
   1. ask the patient to demonstrate the technique on a tooth model
   2. have the patient floss his or her entire mouth for you
   3. evaluate the amount of deposits and the condition of the patient's gingiva at the next appointment
   4. have the patient explain the flossing procedure to you just as you have explained it to the patient

7. **2A** Which of the following is the most successful approach to caries prevention in the general population?
  1. regular recall appointments
  2. the use of fluorides
  3. nutritional education
  4. flossing and brushing

8. **2A** After determining the need for nutritional counseling, which of the following are essential components of the process?
  (a) determining the patient's current food consumption
  (b) determining the reasons for the current status of the diet
  (c) putting the patient on a sucrose-free diet
  (d) working with the patient to change nutritional habits
  1. (a), (b) and (c)
  2. (a), (b) and (d)
  3. (b), (c) and (d)
  4. All of the above

9. **2A** Which of the following have been demonstrated to be the most successful approach to preventing periodontal disease in the general population?
  (a) the use of fluorides
  (b) nutritional education
  (c) flossing and brushing
  (d) regular recall appointments
  1. (a), (b) and (c)
  2. (b), (c) and (d)
  3. (b) and (d) only
  4. (c) and (d) only
  5. All of the above

10. **1A** Caries occurs most often during a time when the pH of the plaque is
  1. above 9
  2. 7
  3. below 5
  4. None of the above

11. **3B** When providing nutritional counseling, instructing patients to follow the "Basic Four" approach means
  1. ensuring that they are acquiring the R.D.A. in all nutrients
  2. providing that they have the minimum necessary proteins and carbohydrates
  3. that it is recommended by the F.D.A.
  4. All of the above

12. **1A** The patient who smokes needs higher daily amounts of vitamin
  1. A
  2. B
  3. C
  4. D
  5. All of the above (Smoking affects the body's reserves of vitamins and minerals.)

13. **1A** Cheilosis is the manifestation of a deficiency in
  1. vitamin C
  2. protein
  3. niacin
  4. riboflavin

14. **2A** Which of the following nutrient's is lacking in nonfortified skimmed milk?
  1. calcium
  2. riboflavin
  3. phosphorus
  4. vitamin D

15. **2A** Vitamin C in foods is destroyed by
  1. cooking for long periods of time
  2. leaving foods stored open in the refrigerator
  3. exposure to alkalies
  4. All of the above

16. Which of the following are considered
2A food sources from the meat group of
the "Basic Four"?
    (a) chicken
    (b) fish
    (c) nuts
    (d) legumes
  1. (a), (b) and (c)
  2. (a) and (b) only
  3. (b), (c) and (d)
  4. (b) and (c) only
  5. All of the above

17. If a patient is on a cholesterol-restric-
3B tive diet, which of the following should
not be recommended as part of that
diet?
    (a) liver
    (b) eggs
    (c) shellfish
    (d) skimmed milk
  1. (a), (b) and (c)
  2. (a) and (b) only
  3. (b), (c) and (d)
  4. (b) and (c) only
  5. All of the above

18. A deficiency of nicotinic acid (niacin)
1A may result in
    (a) dark, scaly dermatitis
    (b) glossitis
    (c) pellagra
    (d) loss of appetite
  1. (a) and (b)
  2. (b), (c) and (d)
  3. (b) only
  4. (c) only
  5. All of the above

19. A yellow color in plants indicates the
3B presence of
  1. vitamin C
  2. vitamin A
  3. phosphorus
  4. vitamin E

20. No milk products should be taken
1A within 45 minutes of ingestion of the
drug
  1. penicillin
  2. ampicillin
  3. tetracycline
  4. sulfa

21. The M.D.R. (Minimum Daily Re-
3B quirement) is
    (a) set by the Food and Drug Ad-
ministration
    (b) synonymous with the R.D.A
    (c) used in labeling
    (d) a measure of the quantities of
nutrients necessary for health
  1. (a), (b) and (c)
  2. (a) and (c) only
  3. (b) and (c) only
  4. (b) and (d) only
  5. All of the above

22. When providing nutritional counseling
3B for a child patient with frequent caries,
it should be stressed that
  1. sucrose is the only sugar that
causes caries
  2. the more sugar in a food, the more
cariogenic its potential
  3. the frequency of ingesting sugar is
the most important consideration
  4. All of the above

23. Dentin may become exposed through
1A 1. improper toothbrushing technique
  2. cervical caries
  3. root planing
  4. All of the above

24. When evaluating a patient's tissue re-
4B sponse to a recommended plaque control program, the most important tool
is
1. disclosing solution
2. periodontal probing
3. the patient's motivation
4. radiographs

25. Which of the following should be in-
1A cluded in a preventive program de-
or signed for an 8-year-old boy with sev-
3B eral carious lesions?
(a) education of the parent as to
the relationship between
plaque and caries
(b) a regular fluoride program
(c) nutritional counseling
(d) toothbrushing instruction only,
because of the patient's age
1. (a), (b) and (c)
2. (a), (b) and (d)
3. (a) and (b)
4. (b) and (d)
5. All of the above

26. When instructing a patient in the use
3B of dental floss, it should be stressed
that
(a) floss should be used once a
day
(b) flossing should be performed
before brushing
(c) only unwaxed floss should be
used
1. (a) and (b) only
2. (b) and (c) only
3. All of the above

27. When providing nutritional counseling
3B for a geriatric patient, motivation will
come through
(a) the maintenance of health
(b) the decreased susceptibility to
caries
(c) stressing independence
(d) an expression of concern on the
part of the hygienist
1. (a), (b) and (c)
2. (a), (b) and (d)
3. (a) and (b) only
4. (a), (c) and (d)
5. All of the above

28. In order to motivate a patient to
3B change behavior and accept a suggested plaque control program, you
must
(a) provide a complete presentation of everything concerned
in plaque control
(b) provide immediate feedback
(c) allow time for the patient to
practice the techniques demonstrated
(d) appeal to higher levels of motivation
1. (a), (b) and (c)
2. (a) and (b)
3. (b), (c) and (d)
4. (b) and (c)
5. All of the above

29. After removal, dental plaque that can
2A be detected by disclosing solution reforms
   1. after the next meal
   2. in 8 hours
   3. in 12–24 hours
   4. in 48 hours

30. Video tapes and other forms of self-
2A instructional materials serve which of
the following purposes in a dental office?
   1. teach patients how to brush and
      floss
   2. establish in the patient a value for
      good dental health
   3. demonstrate a variety of brushing
      techniques from which to choose
   4. introduce the concept of a per-
      sonal plaque control program

31. If a patient receives plaque control in-
4A structions, including flossing technique, from a dental hygienist and has
two interproximal carious lesions at the
next recall appointment, the dental hygienist should conclude
   1. the patient did not floss
   2. the patient's sucrose intake is too
      high
   3. flossing did not prevent dental car-
      ies
   4. All of the above
   5. None of the above

32. Acquired pellicle reforms
4A 1. 24 hours after flossing and brush-
      ing
   2. almost immediately after flossing
      and brushing
   3. after the next food ingestion im-
      mediately following cleaning of
      the teeth
   4. None of the above

33. Dentifrices approved by the American
2A Dental Association must
   1. act as a detergent in cleaning the
      teeth
   2. disrupt the oral flora inhibiting
      cariogenic conditions
   3. aid in increasing enamel resistance
      to acid
   4. None of the above

34. Dental caries is caused by
2A 1. plaque
   2. calculus
   3. carbohydrates
   4. All are equally responsible.

35. Greene and Vermillion's OHI-S mea-
1A sures
   1. decay
   2. periodontal disease
   3. missing teeth
   4. debris

36. Gingival inflammation can be mea-
1A sured by
or   (a) the presence of bleeding
4B   (b) the color of the papillary and
         marginal areas
      (c) monitoring gingival crevicular
         fluid
   1. (a), (b) and (c)
   2. (a) and (b) only
   3. (a) and (c) only
   4. (b) and (c) only

37. The body stores carbohydrates in the
2A muscles and liver in the form of
   1. glucose
   2. glycogen
   3. pectins
   4. dextrins

65

38. The streptocci in the oral cavity which
1A contribute to caries activity are strep-
tococci
    (a) mutans
    (b) viridans
    (c) sanguis
    (d) hemolytic
    1. (a), (b), (c) and (d)
    2. (a) and (c) only
    3. (b) and (d) only
    4. (c) and (d) only

39. After ingestion of a sugar-containing
2A food, microorganisms in the oral cavity
begin acid production after a period
of
    1. 20 minutes
    2. 30 minutes
    3. 1 hour
    4. 30 seconds

40. When providing nutritional counsel-
2A ing, it should be stressed that this caries inducing acid production
    1. lasts approximately 20 minutes
    2. lasts approximately 8 hours
    3. lasts until the next meal
    4. is of very limited duration due to
    the buffering action of the saliva,
    which recovers to basic almost im-
    mediately

41. Oral irrigation devices are important in
2A a personal oral hygiene program because the action of the water
    1. dislodges food debris from orth-
    odontic bands
    2. dislodges loosened debris from
    under pontics
    3. removes plaque from the proximal
    surfaces of the teeth
    4. both (1) and (2)
    5. both (1) and (3)

42. When using an oral irrigation device,
3B the patient should be instructed to
    1. use the device on the highest set-
    ting
    2. point the head of the device to-
    ward the apex of the tooth
    3. use the device to flush out the gin-
    gival sulcus
    4. point the device straight on be-
    tween the proximal surfaces
    5. All of the above are useful tech-
    niques when using the device.

43. Cellulose is a polysaccharide synthe-
2A sized from parts of plants that
    1. is stored in the body in the liver
    and muscle tissues
    2. is not digestible by humans
    3. aids in the stimulation of peristal-
    sis and the elimination of waste
    4. only (1) and (3)
    5. only (2) and (3)

44. Body proteins are broken down into
2A essential amino acids through the met-
abolic function of
    1. anabolism
    2. catabolism
    3. enzymization
    4. protein synthesis

45. Which is the hormone that stimulates
1A the digestive process of fats in the
or small intestine?
2A 1. bile
    2. cholcystokinin
    3. gastrin
    4. pepsin

46. The process of protein digestion begins
1A in the
or 1. mouth
2A 2. stomach
    3. small intestine
    4. large intestine

47. The pregnant patient needs increased
1A amounts of which of the following?
    (a) iron
    (b) calcium
    (c) vitamin D
    (d) sodium
    1. (a), (b) and (c)
    2. (a), (b) and (d)
    3. (a) and (b) only
    4. (b) and (c) only
    5. All of the above

48. When instructing a patient in sulcular
3B toothbrushing technique, which of the
    following should be included?
    1. use of a soft, multitufted tooth-
       brush
    2. instruction in angulation of the
       brush toward the occlusal sur-
       faces
    3. a brush with rounded bristles
    4. (1) and (2)
    5. (1) and (4) only

49. The Modified Stillman toothbrushing
3B technique
    1. is recommended for children
    2. is designed for massage and stimu-
       lation as well as cleaning
    3. is accomplished by angulation of
       the bristles toward the occlusal
    4. utilizes a circular motion of the
       bristles

50. When providing toothbrushing in-
3B structions for a young child, which of
    the following should be recom-
    mended?
    (a) a soft toothbrush
    (b) the Fones brushing technique
    (c) the Bass brushing technique
    (d) a vibratory stroke
    1. (a) and (b)
    2. (a), (c) and (d)
    3. (a) and (c)
    4. (c) and (d)

Chapter 7

Providing Supportive Treatment Services

Providing *support services* to the dentist throughout a dental procedure is a key function of the dental hygienist. On the National Board Examination there are 46 questions devoted to various support services, which include asepsis and sterilization, pain control, polishing restorations and margination, and other support services. This last area is quite broad, as evidenced in the chart. Sixteen questions are allotted to it on the Examination; hence, a variety of questions are included here. Because most states allow dental hygienists to place cements, bases, a matrix band and wedge, and to apply rubber dams, major emphasis is placed on these items. Since few states authorize hygienists to place permanent (alloy and composition) restorations or to inject local anesthetics, the number of questions relating to these items is limited.

Function	Questions and Categories
1. Asepsis and sterilization	11 questions 6-**A**; 3-**B**; 2-**C**
2. Pain control	9 questions - **A**
3. Polishing restorations and removing excess restorative materials	10 questions 6-**A**; 2-**B**; 2-**C**
4. Other supportive services (i.e., removing sutures, placing and removing surgical dressings, placing and removing temporary restorations	16 questions 8-**A**; 4-**B**; 4-**C**

A-background information
B-methodology
C-armamentarium

Recommended References

American Dental Association. *Accepted dental therapeutics*. Chicago: 1982.

Crawford, J., et al. Suggested guidelines for asepsis in the dental office environment. *Dental Hygiene*, Oct. 1981.

Pattison, G. and Pattison, A. *Periodontal instrumentation*. Reston, Va.: Reston Publishing, 1979.

Philips, R. *Elements of dental materials*. Philadelphia: Saunders, 1977.

Project Accorde. *Restorations of cavity preparations with amalgam and tooth colored materials*. Castro Valley, Calif.: Quercus, 1978.

Wheeler, R. *Dental anatomy*. Philadelphia: Saunders, 1974.

Wilkins, E. *Clinical practice of the dental hygienist*. Philadelphia: Lea & Febiger, 1983.

Woodall, I., et al. *Comprehensive dental hygiene care*. St. Louis: C. V. Mosby, 1980.

Questions

1.
3A Contraindication(s) for the removal of
excess amalgam is (are)
  1. presence of recurrent decay
  2. fracture line
  3. open contact
  4. too large an overhang
  5. All of the above

2.
4B When placing a rubber dam using a
wingless clamp, you should perform
the following steps in what order?
  (a) relate punched holes to corre-
sponding teeth
  (b) ease interseptal dam material
through contacts
  (c) slip dam over the bow of the
clamp and then each jaw
  (d) isolate the most anterior teeth
  1. (a), (b), (c), (d)
  2. (a), (c), (b), (d)
  3. (b), (d), (a), (c)
  4. (c), (d), (a), (b)
  5. (d), (a), (b), (c)

3.
4A On the maxillary molars, the groove
that extends from the posterior of the
chewing surface to the lingual of the
tooth is called the
  1. mesio-occlusal groove
  2. occlusolingual groove
  3. distolingual groove
  4. secondary central groove

4.
2A You are going to do soft tissue curettage on 29–31 on the facial tissue only.
What injection would be indicated?
  1. inferior alveolar
  2. lingual
  3. long buccal
  4. papillary

5.
4B In removing continuous sutures, the
operator
  (a) cuts between the knot and tissue
  (b) cuts the vertical loops of the
suture interproximally facially
and lingually
  (c) removes the continuous suture
by withdrawing its entire
length
  (d) withdraws strands that have
been clipped into pieces
  1. (a), (b) and (c)
  2. (a), (b) and (d)
  3. (a), (c) and (d)
  4. (b), (c) and (d)
  5. None of the above

6.
1A Your patient is a hepatitis B carrier.
Proper handling procedure of your instruments after you have completed
treatment would be to
  1. wash, scrub, ultrasonic, and sterilize
  2. sterilize, ultrasonic, and sterilize
  3. ultrasonic, wash/scrub, and sterilize
  4. scrub with iodine then sterilize

7.
2A The following is a common vasocon-
strictor used in local anesthesia:
  1. epinephrine
  2. norepinephrine
  3. levonordefrin
  4. mepivacaine hydrochloride (Car-
bocaine)

8.
4B The rubber dam clamp should be
placed securely
  1. on the enamel
  2. apical to the cervical contour
  3. apical to the margin of the free gingiva
  4. in the gingiva, if necessary, to stabilize the clamp

71

9. Overhangs can be detected
3B   1. visually
  2. tactilely
  3. radiographically
  4. All of the above
  5. None of the above

10. Improper placement of a wedge could
4A cause
  (a) open contacts
  (b) displacement of the matrix band during condensing
  (c) overhangs
  (d) increased height of the marginal ridge
  1. (a), (b) and (c)
  2. (a), (b) and (d)
  3. (b), (c) and (d)
  4. (a), (c) and (d)
  5. All of the above

11. Which of the following are typical of
2A nitrous oxide sedation?
  (a) Effects are rapidly produced.
  (b) Effects are easily regulated by changing the mixture.
  (c) Effects are rapidly reversed by supplying pure oxygen.
  (d) The patient is relaxed and the pain threshold is often raised.
  1. (a), (b) and (c)
  2. (a), (c) and (d)
  3. (b), (c) and (d)
  4. All of the above
  5. None of the above

12. Once excess amalgam has been re-
3B moved, the interproximal area must be
  1. polished until it is no longer plaque retentive
  2. polished through the contact with a finishing strip
  3. smoothed with a green stone
  4. smoothed with a high-speed bur

13. Vasoconstrictors are contraindicated in
2A patients who have
  (a) hyperthyroidism
  (b) cardiac arrhythmias
  (c) hypertension
  (d) prolonged bleeding
  1. (a), (b) and (c)
  2. (a), (c) and (d)
  3. (b), (c) and (d)
  4. All of the above
  5. None of the above

14. Instrument packs that have been ster-
1A ilized should be dated. Unused packs should be reprocessed after
  1. 2 weeks
  2. 4 weeks
  3. 6 weeks
  4. 2 months

15. Marginal ridges are found on which of
4A the following teeth?
  1. anterior
  2. posterior
  3. molars
  4. all teeth

16. Types of periodontal packs include
4C   (a) mixtures with eugenol
  (b) mixtures without eugenol
  (c) plastics (cyanoacrylates)
  (d) zinc phosphate
  1. (a), (b) and (c)
  2. (a), (c) and (d)
  3. (b), (c) and (d)
  4. All of the above
  5. None of the above

17. If a deficiency has been created (too
3B much amalgam removed), the explorer will
  1. catch when passed from tooth to amalgam
  2. catch when passed from amalgam to tooth
  3. catch when passed both ways
  4. click in both directions

18. The patient has a history of liver dis-
2A ease. You would choose an anesthetic
    that is *not*
    1. an amide type
    2. an ester type
    3. combined with a vasoconstrictor
    4. combined with a vasodilator

19. Proper timing for the autoclave steril-
1B ization cycle should begin
       (a) when the door is properly
           sealed
       (b) after the proper temperature is
           reached
       (c) after the proper pressure is
           reached
       (d) after 15 minutes
    1. (a), (b) and (c)
    2. (a), (c) and (d)
    3. (b), (c) and (d)
    4. All of the above
    5. None of the above

20. When placing a rubber dam clamp, the
4B clamp is usually placed *first* on the
    1. lingual then the facial
    2. facial then the lingual
    3. lingual, and it will then slip into
       place on the facial
    4. facial, and it will then slip into
       place on the lingual

21. Normally, after the administration of
2A nitrous oxide, the patient should
    1. breathe 6–8 liters of pure oxygen
       for at least 5 minutes
    2. breathe 6–8 liters of pure oxygen
       for at least 10 minutes
    3. not be allowed to drive home
    4. be given an ammonia inhalant

22. The purpose of using a wooden wedge
4C is to
    1. separate the teeth to allow for
       proximal contact
    2. stabilize the matrix band
    3. prevent overhangs
    4. All of the above
    5. None of the above

23. The proper sequence for removing a
4B rubber dam is to
       (a) remove the clamp
       (b) cut the interseptal portions of
           the dam with scissors
       (c) remove the dam
       (d) unfasten the dam holder
    1. (a), (b), (c), (d)
    2. (a), (b), (d), (c)
    3. (b), (a), (c), (d)
    4. (b), (a), (d), (c)

24. When removing a Tofflemire matrix
4B retainer band, you should remove
    the
    1. band first
    2. retainer first
    3. band and retainer together
    4. band *or* retainer first, whichever is
       easier

25. Which of the following acts primarily
2A in the central nervous system?
    1. nitrous oxide
    2. local anesthetic
    3. topical anesthetic
    4. spray lidocaine

26. Gingival overhangs are the result of
3A
1. inadequate condensing
2. condensing too forcefully in the proximal box
3. excessive tightening of the matrix band
4. improper use of the wooden wedge

27. The proximal contact area of a Class II
4A restoration should be
1. in the incisal/occlusal one-third of the tooth
2. between the incisal/occlusal one-third and the middle third of the tooth
3. in the middle third of the tooth
4. between the middle third and the gingival one-third of the tooth

28. As a precaution when utilizing the
1B high-speed handpiece or ultrasonic (cavitron) scaler, you should wear
1. gloves, mask and eye cover
2. mask and eye cover
3. bib, gloves and eye cover
4. gloves and eye cover

29. The patient has pulmonary disease.
2A Which of the following pain control procedures is contraindicated?
1. local anesthetic
2. topical anesthetic
3. tranquilizers
4. nitrous oxide - oxygen

30. A rubber dam is used to
4A
1. maintain a dry field
2. prevent aspiration and swallowing of foreign objects
3. allow for improved visibility
4. All of the above

31. Periodontal dressings can be used in
4A procedures such as
(a) gingivectomy
(b) gingivoplasty
(c) mucogingival surgery
(d) soft tissue curettage
1. (a), (b) and (c)
2. (a), (c) and (d)
3. (b), (c) and (d)
4. All of the above
5. None of the above

32. When polishing the finished restora-
3B tion, the purpose of using water in the polishing compound is to
1. bring a greater luster to the amalgam
2. prevent rapid tarnishing of the amalgam
3. reduce the heat generated by the cup or brush
4. make the polishing agent easier to use

33. A periodontal pack is
4B
(a) applied to facial portions of the wound
(b) applied to lingual portions of the wound
(c) connected interproximally
(d) applied occlusally beyond the height of contour
1. (a), (b) and (c)
2. (a), (c) and (d)
3. (b), (c) and (d)
4. All of the above
5. None of the above

34. When preparing a matrix for a Class II
4A temporary restoration, what determines if a wedge is placed from the buccal or lingual? The size of the
1. occlusal embrasure
2. wedge
3. restoration
4. gingival embrasure

35. The proper aseptic procedure to follow
1B after using rubber prophylaxis cups
and brushes is
 (a) using a gas or steam autoclave
 (b) discarding them
 (c) scrubbing and soaking them in alcohol
 (d) wrapping them in Cidex
 1. (a) and (b) only
 2. (b) and (c) only
 3. (c) and (d) only
 4. All of the above
 5. None of the above

36. In preparing the temporary restoration
4B of a Class II mesio-occlusal with zinc
oxide-eugenol
 1. excursive contact should be present
 2. centric contact should be present
 3. protrusive contact should be present
 4. the temporary restoration should be slightly over-carved

37. The advantage of a polished amalgam
3A over an unpolished one is that it
 1. is easier to clean
 2. resists tarnish and corrosion
 3. will have less marginal deterioration
 4. All of the above

38. The proximal surface of an amalgam
3B restoration is best polished by
 1. a linen finishing strip
 2. waxed dental tape and pumice
 3. a diamond strip
 4. a green stone
 5. the EVA system

39. Which of the following is a function of a
4C matrix? It
 1. establishes proper anatomic contour
 2. keeps the operating field clear and dry
 3. enhances access to the cavity preparation
 4. separates the teeth

40. The best aseptic procedure in caring
1A for the air/water syringe is to
 1. remove and sterilize it like an instrument
 2. soak gauze in alcohol and then wrap the syringe with it
 3. remove it and place it in disinfectant
 4. spray it for 15 seconds before wrapping it in alcohol-soaked gauze.

41. A periodontal pack must be adapted to
4B the tissue. The following can be used:
 (a) the back of a curette
 (b) a cotton swab
 (c) pliers
 (d) Black's gold knife
 1. (a), (b) and (c)
 2. (a), (c) and (d)
 3. (b), (c) and (d)
 4. All of the above
 5. None of the above

42. Recent evidence indicates that there is
2A an increased rate of miscarriage among
female patients and female dental personnel who have been exposed to
 1. local anesthetics in the first trimester
 2. nitrous oxide
 3. pure oxygen in the first trimester
 4. ultrasound in excess of 20,000 cycles

75

43. After attempting to remove excess
3B amalgam, the margin should be
    checked with an explorer. If there is
    still excess, the explorer will
    1. catch when passed from tooth to
       amalgam
    2. catch when passed from amalgam
       to tooth
    3. catch when passed both ways
    4. click in both directions

44. The instrument of choice for a me-
3C dium-size overhang is a
    1. gracey curette
    2. gold-knife
    3. hoe
    4. finishing file

45. Temporary restorations are made of
4A zinc oxide-eugenol instead of zinc
    phosphate because ZOE
    1. has an irritating effect on the
       pulp
    2. is more esthetically pleasing
    3. though weaker, is easier to re-
       move
    4. is stronger and easier to remove

46. The action of the following pieces of
1A equipment can suck back saliva and
    thereby cause contamination:
    (a) pulp tester
    (b) air/water syringe
    (c) high-speed handpiece
    (d) cavitron
    1. (a) and (b) only
    2. (b) and (c) only
    3. (c) and (d) only
    4. All of the above
    5. None of the above

47. A zinc oxide temporary restoration can
4A remain in the tooth as long as
    1. 2 weeks
    2. 6 weeks
    3. 2 months
    4. 6 months

48. To determine if a matrix band is ex-
4B tended adequately in an occlusal direc-
    tion, compare it with the marginal
    ridge of the
    1. adjacent tooth
    2. same tooth on the opposite side of
       the arch
    3. same tooth in the opposite arch
    4. All of the above

49. The purpose of polishing amalgams is
3A to
    1. remove scratches, pits and flash
    2. remove excess mercury
    3. create a shiny restoration
    4. All of the above
    5. None of the above

50. When placing a rubber dam, the clamp
4C of choice
    (a) adapts to the contours of the
        tooth
    (b) does not impinge unnecessar-
        ily
    (c) is always placed on the enamel
        surface
    (d) can be stabilized with dental
        floss
    (e) can be rocked slightly buccol-
        ingually with the fingers
    1. (a), (b) and (c)
    2. (a) only
    3. (a) and (b) only
    4. All of the above

51. A wooden wedge should be placed so
4B that the base of the triangle is toward
the
1. buccal
2. gingival
3. mesial or distal
4. occlusal

52. When restoring a Class IV mesioincisal
4A cavity preparation, you must recreate
   (a) the incisal angle
   (b) part of the mesial marginal
       ridge
   (c) part of the proximal surface
   (d) part of the facial surface
1. (a), (b), (c) and (d)
2. (a), (c), and (d)
3. (a) and (c)
4. (b), (c) and (d)

53. Hepatitis B is most frequently trans-
1B mitted through
   (a) blood
   (b) saliva
   (c) semen
   (d) feces
1. (a), (b) and (c)
2. (a), (c) and (d)
3. (b), (c) and (d)
4. All of the above
5. None of the above

54. The major part of the dental anatomy
4A with which to be concerned when carving a Class V restoration on the buccal
of the mandibular right first molar is
the
1. proximal embrasure
2. facial groove
3. distobuccal groove
4. Carabelli cusp

55. While wearing a periodontal pack, the
4A patient is advised
1. *not* to brush the dressing
2. to brush and floss the rest of the
   mouth as usual
3. to rinse with warm water four
   times a day
4. All of the above
5. None of the above

56. After placement of a periodontal pack,
4A the patient should return to have it
removed in
1. 2–3 days
2. 3–4 days
3. 5–7 days
4. 7–10 days

57. In polishing and finishing alloys, the
3B final agent to be used is
1. zinc oxide and eugenol
2. whiting (calcium carbonate)
3. tin oxide
4. pumice

58. After a periodontal pack is removed,
4B the area is rinsed with
1. a pulsating water lavage device
2. an air/water syringe
3. salt water
4. an oxygenating agent

59. A patient enters the office complaining
2A of pain in tooth number 12. The dentist
decides to anesthetize in order to exca-
vate the caries. The following injection
will most likely be performed:
1. middle superior alveolar
2. posterior superior alveolar
3. infraorbital
4. greater palatine

60. The minimum amount of time that
3A must elapse after carving the amalgam restoration and before beginning the finishing and polishing procedures is
   1. 12 hours
   2. 24 hours
   3. 36 hours
   4. 48 hours

61. In removing a periodontal dressing,
4B sutures are sometimes caught in the dressing. The proper procedure is which of the following?
   1. Break the dressing into pieces, leaving the area with sutures intact.
   2. If the sutures are tied on the facial, remove the lingual portion first.
   3. If the sutures are tied on the facial, remove the facial portion first.
   4. Gently cut through the pack and then cut the suture knot.

62. Water steam sterilization (autoclave) is
1B effective at
   1. 121°C/15 lbs./15–20 min.
   2. 120°F/15 lbs./30 min.
   3. 350°F/20 lbs./25 min.
   4. 121°C/15 lbs./5–10 min.

63. The purpose of a peridontal dressing is
4A to
   (a) protect the surgical area
   (b) promote healing
   (c) stabilize mobile teeth
   (d) protect sutures
   (e) help control bleeding
   (f) help protect sensitive teeth from temperature changes
   1. (a), (b), (c), (d) and (e)
   2. (a), (c), (d), (e) and (f)
   3. (b), (c), (d), (e) and (f)
   4. All of the above
   5. None of the above

64. Polishing order is reflected in the use
3B of materials from course to fine. The following would be an example:
   1. medium cuttle disks, strips, pumice, tin oxide
   2. strips, medium cuttle disks, pumice, tin oxide
   3. pumice, medium cuttle disks, strips, tin oxide
   4. tin oxide, medium cuttle disks, strips, pumice

65. Proper dry heat sterilization is
1C 1. 150°C for 90 minutes
   2. 160°F for 60 minutes
   3. 160–170°C for 60 minutes
   4. 350°C for 30 minutes

66. Which of the following are *not* recom-
1A mended for disinfecting instruments and surfaces used in dentistry?
   (a) 90% isopropanol
   (b) 90% ethanol
   (c) 1–3% phenolics
   (d) quaternary ammonium compounds
   1. (a), (b) and (c)
   2. (a), (c) and (d)
   3. (b), (c) and (d)
   4. All of the above
   5. None of the above

67. In removing interrupted sutures of a
4B periodontal pack, the operator
   1. pulls gently on the knot and cuts the suture between the knot and the tissue
   2. pulls the knotted end through the tissue
   3. cuts the suture on the tooth surface opposite the knot
   4. uses a sickle scaler to cut the suture

Chapter 8

Assisting in Emergencies

There is always a chance that an emergency will arise in the course of a complicated procedure or even during the most routine dental appointment. In order to best assist the dentist, the hygienist must be able to recognize potential situations and signs of emergencies. Knowledge of remedial techniques to be used in particular emergency situations and maintenance of the armamentarium can help to bring an emergency quickly under control. The 28 questions in this section of the National Board Examination stress the importance of adequate background information and familiarity with methods and the armamentarium.

Function	Questions and Categories
1. Recognizing the potential for emergency situations	9 questions **A**
2. Recognizing an emergency situation	8 questions - **A**
3. Providing emergency care	11 questions 9-**B**; 2-**C**

A-background information
B-methodology
C-armamentarium

Recommended References

American Dental Association. *Accepted dental therapeutics*. Chicago, 1982.

Malamud, S. *Handbook of local anesthesia*. St. Louis: C. V. Mosby, 1980.

Wilkins, E. *Clinical practice of the dental hygienist*. Philadelphia: Lea & Febiger, 1983.

Woodall, I., et al. *Comprehensive dental hygiene care*. St. Louis: C. V. Mosby, 1980.

Questions

1. In attempting to dislodge a foreign ob-
3B ject from an unconscious victim, you
would
   1. apply blows to the back, apply an
abdominal thrust, and remove the
object with your finger
   2. administer oxygen
   3. apply an abdominal thrust, apply
blows to the back, and remove the
object with your finger
   4. None of the above

2. You come upon an unconscious victim
2A whose pupils are dilated and who has
no pulse or heart beat. This condition
has most likely been present for at
least
   1. 1½ minutes
   2. 50 seconds
   3. 30 seconds
   4. 10 seconds

3. Hyperventilation is characterized by
2A (a) rapid breathing
   (b) acute anxiety
   (c) tingling or numbness in fingers
   (d) lower blood pressure
   1. (a), (b) and (c)
   2. (a), (c) and (d)
   3. (b), (c) and (d)
   4. All of the above
   5. None of the above

4. An ambu bag
3C (a) attaches to a portable oxygen
tank system
   (b) is able to force 100% oxygen
into the patient's lungs
   (c) is necessary if a positive pressure oxygen mask is not available
   (d) is important if the patient is
unable to breathe unassisted
   1. (a), (b) and (c)
   2. (a), (b) and (d)
   3. (a), (c) and (d)
   4. (b), (c) and (d)
   5. All of the above

5. Which of the following indicate that
1A the hygienist should anticipate the
possible need for emergency procedures?
   (a) epilepsy
   (b) hepatitis
   (c) diabetes
   (d) angina pectoris
   (e) rheumatic fever
   1. (a), (b) and (c)
   2. (a), (c) and (d)
   3. (a), (c) and (e)
   4. (b), (c) and (d)
   5. (b), (d) and (e)

6. During simple syncope you may see
2A   (a) loss of skin color
      (b) perspiration
'   (c) slight confusion
      (d) muscle twitching
  1. (a), (b) and (c)
  2. (a), (c) and (d)
  3. (b), (c) and (d)
  4. All of the above
  5. None of the above

7. Your patient appears to be having
3B heart failure; as long as the patient is conscious, you should place him or her in an upright position *because* this position allows excess fluid to settle in the lower lung so that there can be some exchange of air in the tissue.
  1. The statement is correct, but the reason is incorrect.
  2. Both the statement and the reason are correct and related.
  3. Both the statement and the reason are correct, but not related.
  4. Neither the statement nor the reason is correct.

8. Bacteremia has been demonstrated fol-
1A lowing
    (a) toothbrushing
    (b) radiography
    (c) scaling
    (d) polishing
  1. (a), (b) and (c)
  2. (a), (c) and (d)
  3. (b), (c) and (d)
  4. All of the above
  5. None of the above

9. Your patient suddenly coughs a bloody
2A sputum and complains of suffocation; cyanosis follows. The most probable cause is
  1. syncope
  2. epilepsy
  3. heart failure
  4. hyperventilation

10. The patient exhibits uncontrolled dia-
1A betes mellitus. Which of the following procedures should be avoided?
    (a) subgingival curettage
    (b) surgery
    (c) placement of a rubber dam
    (d) submarginal probing
  1. (a), (b) and (c)
  2. (a), (c) and (d)
  3. (b), (c) and (d)
  4. All of the above
  5. None of the above

11. The patient has fainted. The order of
3B procedure should be
    (a) Loosen any tight clothing.
    (b) Place a wet towel on the patient's forehead.
    (c) Apply ammonia spirits.
    (d) Lower the patient so that the feet are higher than the head.
  1. (a), (b) and (c)
  2. (a) and (b)
  3. (b), (c) and (d)
  4. (b) and (c)
  5. (d), (a) and (c)

12. The health history notes that the pa-
2A tient takes diphenylhydantoin (Dilantin). During a scaling appointment, the patient loses consciousness. The most probable cause is
  1. syncope
  2. hypoglycemia
  3. hyperventilation
  4. epilepsy

13. You have administered a local anes-
2A thetic. Suddenly the patient experiences edema of the tongue, pharyngeal tissues and larynx. Your patient is experiencing
  1. congestive heart failure
  2. asthmatic attack
  3. anaphylactic reaction
  4. total kidney failure

14. During CPR, the sternum should be
3B compressed
    (a) 1½–2 inches downward in adults
    (b) 2–3 inches downward in adults
    (c) ¾–1½ inches downward in children
    (d) 1½–2 inches downward in children
  1. (a) and (b)
  2. (a) and (c)
  3. (a) and (d)
  4. (b) and (c)
  5. (c) and (d)

15. A patient presents with a history of
1A liver dysfunction. An injection of local anesthetic is indicated. Your choice of anesthetic should be
  1. an ester
  2. an amide
  3. prilocaine hydrochloride (Citanest)
  4. lidocaine hydrochloride (Xylocaine)

16. After cardiac arrest, resuscitation ef-
3B forts must begin immediately because the brain cannot survive without damage for more than
  1. 1–2 minutes
  2. 2–3 minutes
  3. 4–6 minutes
  4. 5–7 minutes

17. Patients with hyperthyroidism should
1A   (a) not be given anesthetic with epinephrine
    (b) not be put under stress
    (c) not be given an ester type anesthetic
    (d) schedule all appointments before noon
  1. (a) and (b)
  2. (a) and (c)
  3. (a) and (d)
  4. (b) and (c)

18. The proper technique of compression
3B to ventilation in two-person CPR is
  1. 15:2
  2. 7:1
  3. 6:1
  4. 5:1

19. When there are situations associated
1A with bacteremia, antibiotic coverage is recommended in the following conditions:
    (a) prosthetic heart valves
    (b) history of rheumatic fever with no rheumatic heart disease
    (c) mitral valve prolapse syndrome
    (d) prosthetic joint replacement
  1. (a), (b) and (c)
  2. (a), (c) and (d)
  3. (b), (c) and (d)
  4. All of the above
  5. None of the above

20. Your patient is having an acute asth-
3B matic attack. You would
    (a) administer oxygen
    (b) spray an epinephrine mist
    (c) apply ammonia salts
    (d) place the patient in a supine position
    1. (a) and (b)
    2. (a) and (c)
    3. (a) and (d)
    4. All of the above
    5. None of the above

21. You have administered three carpules
2A of a local anesthetic as well as a topical subgingival anesthetic. Your patient appears restless, talkative and agitated, and is most probably experiencing
    1. hyperventilation
    2. hyperglycemia
    3. a mild toxic reaction
    4. a severe toxic reaction

22. In patients with a history of angina pec-
1A toris, pain apprehension or excitement should be avoided *because* these factors stimulate the discharge of epinephrine into the circulation, giving rise to increased cardiac rate and blood pressure.
    1. The statement and reason are both correct and related.
    2. The statement is correct, but the reason is not.
    3. The statement and the reason are correct, but unrelated.
    4. The statement and the reason are both incorrect.

23. Your patient is coughing. You notice
3B that the airway seems blocked, and that he or she is having trouble breathing but is able to speak. You would
    1. administer oxygen
    2. apply the Heimlich maneuver
    3. not interfere
    4. place the patient in a supine position

24. Your patient suddenly begins to
2A breathe noisily and shows strain of neck and chest muscles. The most probable cause of this is
    1. syncope
    2. anaphylactic shock
    3. obstruction in the airway
    4. hyperglycemia

25. What ratio of compressions to ventila-
3B tions should a single rescuer use when performing CPR?
    1. 5:1
    2. 5:2
    3. 15:1
    4. 15:2

26. A person with diabetes mellitus should
1A *avoid*
    (a) scheduling an appointment after heavy exercise
    (b) skipping a meal
    (c) scheduling an appointment during the ascending portion of the blood glucose level
    (d) overdosing on insulin
    1. (a), (b) and (c)
    2. (a), (c) and (d)
    3. (b), (c) and (d)
    4. All of the above
    5. None of the above

27. Which of the following are true during
3B the administration of CPR?
    (a) 60–80 compressions/minute in adults
    (b) 100 compressions/minute in children
    (c) Pressure is applied on the top half of the sternum.
    (d) Pressure is applied on the lower sternum.
    1. (a), (b) and (c)
    2. (a), (b) and (d)
    3. (a), (c) and (d)
    4. (b), (c) and (d)
    5. None of the above

28. Your dental hygiene instructor has hy-
3C perventilated. You would
    1. administer epinephrine
    2. have your instructor breathe into a
       plastic bag
    3. place your instructor in a supine
       position
    4. administer oxygen
    5. None of the above

29. During a curettage appointment, you
2A administered a topical anesthetic.
    Later, the patient called to complain of
    a skin rash and itching. This was most
    probably
    1. caused by anaphylactic shock
    2. caused by something unrelated to
       the dental treatment
    3. a mild allergic reaction
    4. caused by contamination during
       the appointment

30. After establishing that the patient is
3B unconscious, the correct procedure to
    follow would be to
    1. place the patient on a hard surface,
       send for help, and open the air-
       way
    2. open the airway, place the patient
       on a hard surface, and send for
       help
    3. send for help, open the airway,
       and place the patient on a hard
       surface
    4. None of the above

31. In patients with cardiac pacemakers,
1A the following may cause adverse ef-
    fects:
    (a) ultrasonic scalers
    (b) pulp testers
    (c) iontophoresis
    (d) motorized dental chairs
    1. (a), (b) and (c)
    2. (a), (c) and (d)
    3. (b), (c) and (d)
    4. All of the above
    5. None of the above

Chapter 9

Participating in Community Health Activities

All dental professionals function within a community to which they can make significant contributions. The dental hygienist is often called upon to assist the community in comparative research and projects designed to promote better dental health. The hygienist must therefore be familiar with both theory and practice in the field of community dentistry in order to fulfill his or her role as a community resource person. In this last section of the National Board Examination, 30 questions are devoted to *community health activities*. They are detailed in the chart.

Function	Questions and Categories
1. Preliminary research	11 questions
a. identifying target population	1-A
b. identifying and measuring factors that influence oral health status	3-A; 3-B
c. establishing channels of communication to promote cooperation	1-A; 1-B
d. determining oral health needs	1-A; 1-B
2. Project planning and operation	10 questions
a. defining project objectives	2-A; 1-B
b. developing project design	1-A; 1-B
c. identifying and gathering resources	1-B
d. selecting appropriate tools and media	1-A; 2-B
e. conducting activity	1-B
3. Project evaluation	9 questions
a. gathering and analyzing project information	1-A; 2-B
b. comparing project results with preliminary data	1-A; 2-B
c. determining the extent to which project objectives were achieved	2-A; 1-B

A-background information   **B**-methodology   **C**-armamentarium

Recommended References

Cormier, P. P., and Levy, J. I. *Community oral health: a systems approach for the dental health profession*. New York: Appleton-Century-Crofts, 1981.

Darby, M. L., and Bowen, D. M. *Research methods for oral health professionals*. St. Louis: C. V. Mosby, 1980.

Dunning, J. M. *Principles of dental public health*. 3rd ed. Cambridge, Mass.: Harvard University Press, 1979.

Jong, A., ed. *Dental public health and community dentistry*. St. Louis: C. V. Mosby, 1981.

Silberman, S. L., and Tryon, A. F. *Community dentistry: a problem-oriented approach*. Littleton, Mass.: PSG Publishing, 1980.

U.S. Dept. of Health, Education, and Welfare, PHS National Institute of Health. *Preventing tooth decay: a guide for implementing self-applied fluoride in schools*. DHEW Publication No. (NIH) 77-1196.

Young, W. O., and Striffler, D. F. *The dentist, his practice, and his community*. 2nd ed. Philadelphia: W. B. Saunders, 1969.

Questions

Questions 1–11 refer to the following case problem:

Grade school children comprise the largest section of the population in a remote rural community. The fluoride level is 0.4 PPM and there is no central water supply. Because dental manpower in this community is so limited, many residents travel long distances to seek dental care. A dentist and hygienist in a neighboring town have been treating the bulk of the population. Initial screenings by the hygienist have demonstrated many cases of rampant decay among the younger children. Most of the dentist's efforts have been spent in extensive restorative treatment. A school nurse has been aware of the extensive dental needs of this rural community and approached the dentist and hygienist to develop some solution to the problem. They contacted the local health department to inform them of their interest in initiating a fluoride mouth rinse program in the community schools.

1. One of the first steps that must be
1aA taken when initiating a fluoride mouth rinse program is to
   1. locate alternative funding sources
   2. inform the community of the program
   3. gain support of the local dental society
   4. identify the target schools that will participate

2. Which of the following will influence
1bB the planning of the program?
   (a) amount of past dental care received by the children
   (b) community attitude towards public health programs
   (c) parents' motivation for oral health improvement
   (d) severity of dental decay among the children
   1. (a), (b) and (c)
   2. (a) and (c)
   3. (b) and (d)
   4. All of the above

3. Initial DMF scores should be taken
1dA prior to conducting the mouth rinse program because these data
   1. measure the degree of dental health in the schoolchildren
   2. serve as a comparison to postprogram scores
   3. are utilized in the evaluation of the program
   4. All of the above
   5. None of the above

4. The dentist and dental hygienist con-
1cA tacted the local health department in order to
   (a) avoid duplication of any similar existing programs
   (b) establish communication with public health officials
   (c) obtain additional materials for conducting the rinse program
   1. (a), (b) and (c)
   2. (a) and (b)
   3. (a) and (c)
   4. (b) and (c)

5.   The best source of information regard-
2cB   ing the concentration of fluoride in the
      water supply is the
      1.   component dental hygiene associ-
           ation
      2.   local school administrator
      3.   state dental school faculty
      4.   dental director of the state health
           department

6.   Which of the following methods will be
1cB   most successful in obtaining support
      for the fluoride mouth rinse program
      from the school board?
      1.   announcements on the radio
      2.   presentations explaining the pro-
           gram during a board meeting
      3.   posters in each school
      4.   letters mailed directly to individ-
           ual board members

7.   Parental approval of student participa-
2bB   tion in the fluoride mouth rinse pro-
      gram can best be secured through
      1.   returned consent forms
      2.   personal letters to the program
           planners
      3.   telephone calls to the school prin-
           cipals
      4.   statements to the PTA
      5.   All of the above

8.   The major objective of the school fluo-
2aB   ride mouth rinse program is to
      1.   motivate teachers to incorporate
           dental topics in class presenta-
           tions
      2.   reduce the caries rate of the
           schoolchildren
      3.   stimulate toothbrushing activities
           in the classroom
      4.   change flossing habits
      5.   make the local childrens' teeth
           stronger

9.   Personnel who should assist in con-
2cB   ducting the fluoride mouth rinse pro-
      gram on a regular basis include
      1.   school teachers
      2.   school nurses
      3.   parents of the children
      4.   All of the above
      5.   None of the above

10.   Educational aids for in-service training
2dB   for personnel involved in the program
      can be obtained from which of the fol-
      lowing?
      1.   National Health Service Corps
      2.   Indian Health Service
      3.   National Institute of Dental Re-
           search
      4.   Head Start programs
      5.   All of the above

11.   Once the program is initiated, the den-
2eB   tist and hygienist can best utilize their
      time by
      1.   dispensing the rinse solution on a
           weekly basis
      2.   monitoring the mouth rinse pro-
           gram
      3.   providing a prophylaxis to each
           participant
      4.   allowing the program to continue
           independently

12.   After computing an OHI-S index on 67
2bB   sixth grade schoolchildren, the dental
      hygienist computed a mean score of
      2.88 for the group. The best approach
      for the continued improvement of the
      oral health status for this group is to
      1.   review form and function of the
           dentition
      2.   discuss the possiblity of home flu-
           oride mouth rinses with parents
      3.   provide a prophylaxis for every
           child
      4.   initiate a plaque control program
           in the classroom starting with ba-
           sic brushing and flossing

13. The best collection measure for pro-
1dB viding vast amounts of unbiased data is
the
1. survey method
2. interview method
3. direct observation method
4. participant observation method

14. The evaluation component of a public
3cA health program should
1. take place after the development
of the project design
2. identify the dental health status of
a target group
3. measure social and political forces
existing in the community
4. reflect the project goals and objectives

15. In the interest of enhancing dental ser-
1bA vices, a nursing home administration
instituted a mandatory in-service training program for the nurses and aids.
The major goal of this program was to
improve the oral health status of the
residents. A dental hygienist presented information on oral conditions
of the elderly, dental hygiene techniques and denture care. The staff also
viewed a film that supplemented the
presentation. At a follow-up session,
the head nurse indicated that the aids
were still not actively involved in dental care maintenance for the residents.
The reason for this response was most
likely due to
1. the quality of the film shown
2. inadequate funds available for development of a maintenance program
3. the dental hygienist's educational
level
4. the aids' lack of motivation towards dental care

16. At what time during planning should
2bA the design of a preventive dental care
program be developed?
1. prior to assessing community
needs
2. prior to contacting health officials
3. after goals and objectives have
been defined
4. simultaneously with the development of an evaluation mechanism

17. The *least* appropriate materials to uti-
2dA lize for dental health education ses-
sions with pregnant patients' are
1. models of primary teeth
2. caries actively testing kits
3. soft bristle toothbrushes
4. posters of the four food groups
5. pamphlets on periodontal disease

18. The best source of dental educational
2dB materials is
1. the American Dental Association
2. a local service organization
3. the state dental society
4. the Kellogg Foundation

19. Objectives developed for dental health
2aA programs should be
(a) stated in measurable terms
(b) based on the needs of the population
(c) developed prior to target
group identification
1. (a), (b) and (c)
2. (a) and (b)
3. (a) and (c)
4. (b) and (c)

20. **1dA** Which of the following most frequently causes difficulty with utilization of periodontal indices?
1. inadequacy of statistical techniques
2. examiner subjectivity in diagnosis of the disease
3. reliability of patient recall
4. sequencing of periodontal therapy

21. **1bB** The most successful approach for passage of fluoridation legislation would be to initially
1. gain the support of influential leaders
2. notify antifluoridationists of public debates to be held in the community
3. organize consumer groups for rallies
4. distribute pamphlets to residents

22. **1bB** Which of the following could *increase* the demand for dental services by the general population?
   (a) greater perceived need for care
   (b) elimination of cost barriers
   (c) increase in birth rate
   (d) increase in educational level
1. (a), (b) and (c)
2. (a), (b) and (d)
3. (b), (c) and (d)
4. All of the above

23. **1bA** Reimbursement terms can greatly affect dental health in a community. In reimbursement terms, an arrangement where the carrier and beneficiary are each responsible for a portion of the cost of services is referred to as:
1. coinsurance
2. deductible
3. capitation
4. table of allowances

For Questions 24 and 25, refer to the following case:

An experiment was conducted to test the effectiveness of oral hygiene aids, in addition to regular toothbrushing, on oral hygiene status. Seventy-five periodontal patients were randomly distributed into three categories. Participants in Group I were instructed on the use of the proxybrush in addition to regular toothbrushing, Group II received flossing instruction to coincide with brushing. Group III received no additional oral hygiene aids. Plaque and bleeding scores were taken on all participants once every week for a 3-month period.

24. **3aB** Which group served as the control in this study?
1. Group I
2. Group II
3. Group III
4. A control group was *not* utilized in this study.

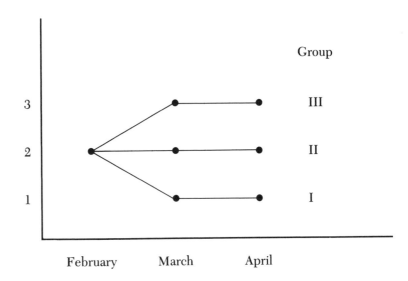

Group

3

Mean plaque
and bleeding
scores

2

1

III

II

I

February   March   April

The results of the experiment described are depicted in the graph above.

25. Additional oral hygiene aids served as
3aB the
1. dependent variable
2. independent variable
3. extraneous variable
4. nonmanipulated variable

26. *What* conclusions may be drawn from
3bB the results as shown on the graph?
   (a) The scores for Group II are invalid
   (b) The proxybrush is a more effective oral hygiene aid than dental floss.
   (c) Plaque and bleeding scores increased in Group III.
   (d) Group II demonstrated *no* change in oral hygiene status during the 3-month period.
1. Both (a) and (b)
2. Both (c) and (d)
3. All of the above

27. The long-range goal of a preventive
2aA dental health education program developed for institutionalized physically handicapped children should be to
1. educate caretakers on basic nutritional concepts
2. train childrens' parents to utilize innovative flossing methods during oral hygiene maintenance
3. motivate children to care for their own oral hygiene needs
4. expose administrators to current research regarding the efficiency of preventive programs for the handicapped

28. A fluoride supplement program was
3cB initiated for preschoolers in a nonfluoridated community. Evaluation of this program after one year should focus on the
1. parents' attitude to the program
2. children's satisfaction with the fluoride solution
3. number of new carious lesions found
4. number of other fluoride programs developed in the community

29.
3bB
A team of dental hygienists determined the initial level of gingivitis among a group of schoolchildren utilizing the gingival index (GI). Five weeks following a program of extensive toothbrushing instruction, 15 dentists scored the same group of subjects. A significant difference existed between the score results due to a lack of calibration among the examiners. The inconsistency occurred because the study lacked

1. interrater reliability
2. intrarater reliability
3. validity
4. sensitivity
5. feasibility

30.
3aA
The following OHI-S scores were obtained during a screening of 56 nursing home residents:

1.76	2.03	2.05	2.56	3.13
1.85	2.04	2.31	2.68	3.13
1.99	2.05	2.56	2.69	3.21

The measure of central tendency that is least useful in analysis of the above data is the

1. mean
2. median
3. mode
4. standard deviation

31.
3bB
Presented in the table are plaque scores of two grades of students involved in a dental health education program.

Mean Plaque Scores

	n	Preprogram	Postprogram
Grade 5	98	2.73	1.80
Grade 7	79	3.54	2.6

Which of the following statements are true?

(a) The difference between preprogram and postprogram scores is the same for both Grades 5 and 7.
(b) The data show an improvement in plaque removal of both grades.
(c) The students in Grade 7 better understood the educational concepts presented in the program.

1. (a) and (b)
2. (a) and (c)
3. (b) and (c)
4. All of the above

32.
1bA
Many factors contribute to individuals not seeking dental care. The barriers with which dental professionals have the most difficulty in effecting change are

1. cognitive barriers
2. psychosocial barriers
3. financial barriers
4. geographic barriers

Answer List

Answers appear in boldface.

Chapter 1: Performing Oral Inspection

1. **3**	11. **1**	21. **3**	30. **2**	39. **3**	48. **3**	57. **4**
2. **1**	12. **1**	22. **2**	31. **4**	40. **1**	49. **1**	58. **1**
3. **4**	13. **4**	23. **3**	32. **5**	41. **1**	50. **5**	59. **5**
4. **2**	14. **4**	24. **4**	33. **3**	42. **5**	51. **1**	60. **4**
5. **4**	15. **4**	25. **3**	34. **1**	43. **3**	52. **2**	61. **2**
6. **2**	16. **3**	26. **1**	35. **3**	44. **4**	53. **3**	62. **2**
7. **2**	17. **3**	27. **3**	36. **2**	45. **2**	54. **4**	63. **5**
8. **5**	18. **4**	28. **2**	37. **1**	46. **5**	55. **4**	64. **3**
9. **2**	19. **5**	29. **3**	38. **1**	47. **1**	56. **4**	65. **3**
10. **4**	20. **1**					

Chapter 2: Exposing and Processing Radiographs

1. **3**	8. **1**	15. **4**	22. **3**	29. **4**	36. **3**	43. **4**
2. **2**	9. **2**	16. **3**	23. **2**	30. **4**	37. **2**	44. **4**
3. **2**	10. **4**	17. **3**	24. **1**	31. **3**	38. **3**	45. **4**
4. **5**	11. **1**	18. **4**	25. **4**	32. **3**	39. **2**	46. **3**
5. **2**	12. **1**	19. **1**	26. **2**	33. **3**	40. **5**	47. **4**
6. **2**	13. **1**	20. **1**	27. **3**	34. **2**	41. **4**	48. **4**
7. **3**	14. **3**	21. **2**	28. **4**	35. **2**	42. **2**	

Chapter 3: Providing Other Diagnostic Aids

1. **1**	6. **2**	11. **3**	16. **1**	21. **3**	26. **3**	31. **3**
2. **1**	7. **4**	12. **1**	17. **2**	22. **3**	27. **2**	32. **5**
3. **3**	8. **2**	13. **1**	18. **2**	23. **4**	28. **3**	33. **4**
4. **1**	9. **3**	14. **4**	19. **2**	24. **3**	29. **4**	34. **4**
5. **2**	10. **2**	15. **4**	20. **3**	25. **2**	30. **3**	35. **2**

Chapter 4: Performing Prophylaxis

1. 3	8. 1	15. 1	21. 2	27. 1	33. 4	39. 3
2. 2	9. 4	16. 3	22. 2	28. 2	34. 2	40. 4
3. 3	10. 3	17. 4	23. 3	29. 2	35. 1	41. 4
4. 2	11. 2	18. 4	24. 4	30. 5	36. 3	42. 4
5. 2	12. 3	19. 1	25. 5	31. 2	37. 1	43. 2
6. 1	13. 1	20. 2	26. 3	32. 5	38. 1	44. 3
7. 2	14. 5					

Chapter 5: Applying Topical Agents

1. 3	5. 4	8. 4	11. 3	14. 3	17. 4	20. 3
2. 3	6. 3	9. 5	12. 3	15. 2	18. 4	21. 3
3. 2	7. 2	10. 4	13. 2	16. 4	19. 3	22. 1
4. 1						

Chapter 6: Providing Individual Oral Health Instruction

1. 4	9. 4	16. 5	23. 4	30. 4	37. 2	44. 2
2. 3	10. 3	17. 1	24. 2	31. 5	38. 2	45. 2
3. 1	11. 2	18. 5	25. 1	32. 2	39. 4	46. 2
4. 4	12. 3	19. 2	26. 1	33. 3	40. 1	47. 1
5. 3	13. 4	20. 3	27. 4	34. 1	41. 4	48. 5
6. 3	14. 4	21. 2	28. 4	35. 4	42. 4	49. 2
7. 2	15. 4	22. 3	29. 3	36. 1	43. 5	50. 1
8. 2						

Chapter 7: Providing Supportive Treatment Services

1. 5	11. 4	21. 1	31. 4	41. 1	50. 3	59. 1
2. 4	12. 1	22. 4	32. 3	42. 2	51. 2	60. 2
3. 3	13. 1	23. 3	33. 1	43. 1	52. 1	61. 2
4. 3	14. 2	24. 2	34. 4	44. 2	53. 1	62. 1
5. 2	15. 4	25. 1	35. 1	45. 3	54. 2	63. 4
6. 2	16. 1	26. 4	36. 4	46. 2	55. 4	64. 1
7. 1	17. 2	27. 2	37. 4	47. 2	56. 3	65. 3
8. 2	18. 1	28. 2	38. 5	48. 1	57. 3	66. 4
9. 4	19. 1	29. 4	39. 1	49. 1	58. 4	67. 1
10. 1	20. 1	30. 4	40. 1			

Chapter 8: Assisting in Emergencies

1. 1	6. 4	11. 5	16. 3	20. 1	24. 3	28. 5
2. 1	7. 2	12. 4	17. 1	21. 3	25. 4	29. 3
3. 1	8. 4	13. 3	18. 4	22. 1	26. 4	30. 1
4. 5	9. 3	14. 2	19. 2	23. 3	27. 2	31. 4
5. 2	10. 4	15. 1				

Chapter 9: Participating in Community Health Activities

1. 4	6. 2	11. 2	16. 3	21. 1	25. 2	29. 1
2. 4	7. 1	12. 4	17. 2	22. 4	26. 2	30. 3
3. 4	8. 2	13. 1	18. 1	23. 1	27. 3	31. 1
4. 1	9. 4	14. 4	19. 2	24. 3	28. 3	32. 2
5. 4	10. 3	15. 4	20. 2			

Practice and Science in Dentistry

quinte//ence books/

Kenneth A. Freedman

Management of the Geriatric Dental Patient

People are living longer; this is inevitably reflected in the composition of the dental practice population. Senior citizens have some oral health problems similar to those of the general population, and other problems that reflect their age and their general health status.

The dentist sees such patients in several settings: his office, homes for the elderly, and—occasionally—in the patient's own home. Each of the settings requires some adaptation if the older patient is to receive care under optimal conditions.

Management of the older patient requires some adjustment on the part of the dentist as well. He must be particularly careful to recognize dental problems associated with long-term use of certain drugs, and he must learn to understand that older patients require special attention. This book will help the concerned dentist to provide optimal care to a growing segment of the population, with minimal disruption of his normal routines.

148 pages, 76 illustrations with 58 in color, size 17.5 × 24.5 cm, linen bound with gold stamping and protective cover.

ISBN 0-931386-05-5

Charles A. Reap, Jr.

Complete Handbook for Dental Auxiliaries

A thinking person's guide to office efficiency and management, Dr. Reap shows auxiliaries how to become stronger members of the dental team, while helping dentists learn to use managerial skills and knowledge to improve practice efficiency. Stressing the importance of "teamwork" and office conferences in avoiding communication breakdown, one re-occurring theme is the auxiliary's responsibility in helping the dentist utilize his or her services and abilities. The auxiliary should be a trouble-shooter, able to anticipate difficulties as well as suggest ways to be of more assistance.

Designed to serve as a post graduate course, this book is divided into four sections which clearly outline the functions of the secretarial assistant, the chairside assistant, the hygienist, and administration of the dental office. Numerous illustrations make the author's thought-provoking suggestions easy to understand and follow. A must for both auxiliary and dentist; it's enlightening for even the most experienced professional.

152 pages, 42 illustrations, size 17.5 × 24.5 cm, soft cover.

ISBN 0-931386-44-6

National Board Examination Answer Sheet

CHAPTER 1

1.
2.
3.
4.
5.
6.
7.
8.
9.
10.
11.
12.
13.
14.
15.
16.
17.
18.
19.
20.
21.
22.
23.
24.
25.
26.
27.
28.
29.
30.
31.
32.
33.
34.
35.
36.
37.
38.
39.
40.
41.
42.
43.
44.
45.
46.
47.
48.
49.
50.
51.
52.
53.
54.
55.
56.
57.
58.
59.
60.
61.
62.
63.
64.
65.

CHAPTER 2

1.
2.
3.
4.
5.
6.
7.
8.
9.
10.
11.
12.
13.
14.
15.
16.
17.
18.
19.
20.
21.
22.
23.
24.
25.
26.
27.
28.
29.
30.
31.
32.
33.
34.
35.
36.
37.
38.
39.
40.
41.
42.
43.
44.
45.
46.
47.
48.

CHAPTER 3

1.
2.
3.
4.
5.
6.
7.
8.
9.
10.
11.
12.
13.
14.
15.
16.
17.
18.
19.
20.
21.
22.
23.
24.
25.
26.
27.
28.
29.
30.
31.
32.
33.
34.
35.

CHAPTER 4

1.
2.
3.
4.
5.
6.
7.
8.
9.
10.
11.
12.
13.
14.
15.
16.
17.
18.
19.
20.
21.
22.
23.
24.
25.
26.
27.
28.
29.
30.
31.
32.
33.
34.
35.
36.
37.
38.
39.
40.
41.
42.
43.
44.

National Board Examination Sheet © 1983
By Quintessence Publishing
Co., Inc. Chicago, Ill.
All Rights Reserved

CHAPTER 5

1. □ □ □ □ □
2. □ □ □ □ □
3. □ □ □ □ □
4. □ □ □ □ □
5. □ □ □ □ □
6. □ □ □ □ □
7. □ □ □ □ □
8. □ □ □ □ □
9. □ □ □ □ □
10. □ □ □ □ □
11. □ □ □ □ □
12. □ □ □ □ □
13. □ □ □ □ □
14. □ □ □ □ □
15. □ □ □ □ □
16. □ □ □ □ □
17. □ □ □ □ □
18. □ □ □ □ □
19. □ □ □ □ □
20. □ □ □ □ □
21. □ □ □ □ □
22. □ □ □ □ □

CHAPTER 6

1. □ □ □ □ □
2. □ □ □ □ □
3. □ □ □ □ □
4. □ □ □ □ □
5. □ □ □ □ □
6. □ □ □ □ □
7. □ □ □ □ □
8. □ □ □ □ □
9. □ □ □ □ □
10. □ □ □ □ □
11. □ □ □ □ □
12. □ □ □ □ □
13. □ □ □ □ □
14. □ □ □ □ □
15. □ □ □ □ □
16. □ □ □ □ □
17. □ □ □ □ □
18. □ □ □ □ □
19. □ □ □ □ □
20. □ □ □ □ □
21. □ □ □ □ □
22. □ □ □ □ □
23. □ □ □ □ □
24. □ □ □ □ □
25. □ □ □ □ □
26. □ □ □ □ □
27. □ □ □ □ □

28. □ □ □ □ □
29. □ □ □ □ □
30. □ □ □ □ □
31. □ □ □ □ □
32. □ □ □ □ □
33. □ □ □ □ □
34. □ □ □ □ □
35. □ □ □ □ □
36. □ □ □ □ □
37. □ □ □ □ □
38. □ □ □ □ □
39. □ □ □ □ □
40. □ □ □ □ □
41. □ □ □ □ □
42. □ □ □ □ □
43. □ □ □ □ □
44. □ □ □ □ □
45. □ □ □ □ □
46. □ □ □ □ □
47. □ □ □ □ □
48. □ □ □ □ □
49. □ □ □ □ □
50. □ □ □ □ □

CHAPTER 7

1. □ □ □ □ □
2. □ □ □ □ □
3. □ □ □ □ □
4. □ □ □ □ □
5. □ □ □ □ □
6. □ □ □ □ □
7. □ □ □ □ □
8. □ □ □ □ □
9. □ □ □ □ □
10. □ □ □ □ □
11. □ □ □ □ □
12. □ □ □ □ □
13. □ □ □ □ □
14. □ □ □ □ □
15. □ □ □ □ □
16. □ □ □ □ □
17. □ □ □ □ □
18. □ □ □ □ □
19. □ □ □ □ □
20. □ □ □ □ □
21. □ □ □ □ □
22. □ □ □ □ □
23. □ □ □ □ □
24. □ □ □ □ □
25. □ □ □ □ □
26. □ □ □ □ □
27. □ □ □ □ □
28. □ □ □ □ □

29. □ □ □ □ □
30. □ □ □ □ □
31. □ □ □ □ □
32. □ □ □ □ □
33. □ □ □ □ □
34. □ □ □ □ □
35. □ □ □ □ □
36. □ □ □ □ □
37. □ □ □ □ □
38. □ □ □ □ □
39. □ □ □ □ □
40. □ □ □ □ □
41. □ □ □ □ □
42. □ □ □ □ □
43. □ □ □ □ □
44. □ □ □ □ □
45. □ □ □ □ □
46. □ □ □ □ □
47. □ □ □ □ □
48. □ □ □ □ □
49. □ □ □ □ □
50. □ □ □ □ □
51. □ □ □ □ □
52. □ □ □ □ □
53. □ □ □ □ □
54. □ □ □ □ □
55. □ □ □ □ □
56. □ □ □ □ □
57. □ □ □ □ □
58. □ □ □ □ □
59. □ □ □ □ □
60. □ □ □ □ □
61. □ □ □ □ □
62. □ □ □ □ □
63. □ □ □ □ □
64. □ □ □ □ □
65. □ □ □ □ □
66. □ □ □ □ □
67. □ □ □ □ □

CHAPTER 8

1. □ □ □ □ □
2. □ □ □ □ □
3. □ □ □ □ □
4. □ □ □ □ □
5. □ □ □ □ □
6. □ □ □ □ □
7. □ □ □ □ □
8. □ □ □ □ □
9. □ □ □ □ □
10. □ □ □ □ □
11. □ □ □ □ □
12. □ □ □ □ □

13. □ □ □ □ □
14. □ □ □ □ □
15. □ □ □ □ □
16. □ □ □ □ □
17. □ □ □ □ □
18. □ □ □ □ □
19. □ □ □ □ □
20. □ □ □ □ □
21. □ □ □ □ □
22. □ □ □ □ □
23. □ □ □ □ □
24. □ □ □ □ □
25. □ □ □ □ □
26. □ □ □ □ □
27. □ □ □ □ □
28. □ □ □ □ □
29. □ □ □ □ □
30. □ □ □ □ □
31. □ □ □ □ □

CHAPTER 9

1. □ □ □ □ □
2. □ □ □ □ □
3. □ □ □ □ □
4. □ □ □ □ □
5. □ □ □ □ □
6. □ □ □ □ □
7. □ □ □ □ □
8. □ □ □ □ □
9. □ □ □ □ □
10. □ □ □ □ □
11. □ □ □ □ □
12. □ □ □ □ □
13. □ □ □ □ □
14. □ □ □ □ □
15. □ □ □ □ □
16. □ □ □ □ □
17. □ □ □ □ □
18. □ □ □ □ □
19. □ □ □ □ □
20. □ □ □ □ □
21. □ □ □ □ □
22. □ □ □ □ □
23. □ □ □ □ □
24. □ □ □ □ □
25. □ □ □ □ □
26. □ □ □ □ □
27. □ □ □ □ □
28. □ □ □ □ □
29. □ □ □ □ □
30. □ □ □ □ □
31. □ □ □ □ □
32. □ □ □ □ □

National Board Examination Answer Sheet

CHAPTER 1

1. 1 2 3 4 5
2. 1 2 3 4 5
3. 1 2 3 4 5
4. 1 2 3 4 5
5. 1 2 3 4 5
6. 1 2 3 4 5
7. 1 2 3 4 5
8. 1 2 3 4 5
9. 1 2 3 4 5
10. 1 2 3 4 5
11. 1 2 3 4 5
12. 1 2 3 4 5
13. 1 2 3 4 5
14. 1 2 3 4 5
15. 1 2 3 4 5
16. 1 2 3 4 5
17. 1 2 3 4 5
18. 1 2 3 4 5
19. 1 2 3 4 5
20. 1 2 3 4 5
21. 1 2 3 4 5
22. 1 2 3 4 5
23. 1 2 3 4 5
24. 1 2 3 4 5
25. 1 2 3 4 5
26. 1 2 3 4 5
27. 1 2 3 4 5
28. 1 2 3 4 5
29. 1 2 3 4 5
30. 1 2 3 4 5
31. 1 2 3 4 5
32. 1 2 3 4 5
33. 1 2 3 4 5
34. 1 2 3 4 5
35. 1 2 3 4 5
36. 1 2 3 4 5
37. 1 2 3 4 5
38. 1 2 3 4 5
39. 1 2 3 4 5
40. 1 2 3 4 5
41. 1 2 3 4 5
42. 1 2 3 4 5
43. 1 2 3 4 5
44. 1 2 3 4 5
45. 1 2 3 4 5
46. 1 2 3 4 5
47. 1 2 3 4 5
48. 1 2 3 4 5
49. 1 2 3 4 5
50. 1 2 3 4 5
51. 1 2 3 4 5
52. 1 2 3 4 5
53. 1 2 3 4 5
54. 1 2 3 4 5
55. 1 2 3 4 5
56. 1 2 3 4 5
57. 1 2 3 4 5
58. 1 2 3 4 5
59. 1 2 3 4 5
60. 1 2 3 4 5
61. 1 2 3 4 5
62. 1 2 3 4 5
63. 1 2 3 4 5
64. 1 2 3 4 5
65. 1 2 3 4 5

CHAPTER 2

1. 1 2 3 4 5
2. 1 2 3 4 5
3. 1 2 3 4 5
4. 1 2 3 4 5
5. 1 2 3 4 5
6. 1 2 3 4 5
7. 1 2 3 4 5
8. 1 2 3 4 5
9. 1 2 3 4 5
10. 1 2 3 4 5
11. 1 2 3 4 5
12. 1 2 3 4 5
13. 1 2 3 4 5
14. 1 2 3 4 5
15. 1 2 3 4 5
16. 1 2 3 4 5
17. 1 2 3 4 5
18. 1 2 3 4 5
19. 1 2 3 4 5
20. 1 2 3 4 5
21. 1 2 3 4 5
22. 1 2 3 4 5
23. 1 2 3 4 5
24. 1 2 3 4 5
25. 1 2 3 4 5
26. 1 2 3 4 5
27. 1 2 3 4 5
28. 1 2 3 4 5
29. 1 2 3 4 5
30. 1 2 3 4 5
31. 1 2 3 4 5
32. 1 2 3 4 5
33. 1 2 3 4 5
34. 1 2 3 4 5
35. 1 2 3 4 5
36. 1 2 3 4 5

CHAPTER 3

1. 1 2 3 4 5
2. 1 2 3 4 5
3. 1 2 3 4 5
4. 1 2 3 4 5
5. 1 2 3 4 5
6. 1 2 3 4 5
7. 1 2 3 4 5
8. 1 2 3 4 5
9. 1 2 3 4 5
10. 1 2 3 4 5
11. 1 2 3 4 5
12. 1 2 3 4 5
13. 1 2 3 4 5
14. 1 2 3 4 5
15. 1 2 3 4 5
16. 1 2 3 4 5
17. 1 2 3 4 5
18. 1 2 3 4 5
19. 1 2 3 4 5
20. 1 2 3 4 5
21. 1 2 3 4 5
22. 1 2 3 4 5
23. 1 2 3 4 5
24. 1 2 3 4 5
25. 1 2 3 4 5
26. 1 2 3 4 5
27. 1 2 3 4 5
28. 1 2 3 4 5
29. 1 2 3 4 5
30. 1 2 3 4 5
31. 1 2 3 4 5
32. 1 2 3 4 5
33. 1 2 3 4 5
34. 1 2 3 4 5
35. 1 2 3 4 5
36. 1 2 3 4 5
37. 1 2 3 4 5
38. 1 2 3 4 5
39. 1 2 3 4 5
40. 1 2 3 4 5
41. 1 2 3 4 5
42. 1 2 3 4 5
43. 1 2 3 4 5
44. 1 2 3 4 5
45. 1 2 3 4 5
46. 1 2 3 4 5
47. 1 2 3 4 5
48. 1 2 3 4 5

CHAPTER 4

1. 1 2 3 4 5
2. 1 2 3 4 5
3. 1 2 3 4 5
4. 1 2 3 4 5
5. 1 2 3 4 5
6. 1 2 3 4 5
7. 1 2 3 4 5
8. 1 2 3 4 5
9. 1 2 3 4 5
10. 1 2 3 4 5
11. 1 2 3 4 5
12. 1 2 3 4 5
13. 1 2 3 4 5
14. 1 2 3 4 5
15. 1 2 3 4 5
16. 1 2 3 4 5
17. 1 2 3 4 5
18. 1 2 3 4 5
19. 1 2 3 4 5
20. 1 2 3 4 5
21. 1 2 3 4 5
22. 1 2 3 4 5
23. 1 2 3 4 5
24. 1 2 3 4 5
25. 1 2 3 4 5
26. 1 2 3 4 5
27. 1 2 3 4 5
28. 1 2 3 4 5
29. 1 2 3 4 5
30. 1 2 3 4 5
31. 1 2 3 4 5
32. 1 2 3 4 5
33. 1 2 3 4 5
34. 1 2 3 4 5
35. 1 2 3 4 5
36. 1 2 3 4 5
37. 1 2 3 4 5
38. 1 2 3 4 5
39. 1 2 3 4 5
40. 1 2 3 4 5
41. 1 2 3 4 5
42. 1 2 3 4 5
43. 1 2 3 4 5
44. 1 2 3 4 5

National Board Examination Sheet © 1983
By Quintessence Publishing
Co., Inc. Chicago, Ill.
All Rights Reserved

CHAPTER 5

1. 2. 3. 4. 5. 6. 7. 8. 9. 10. 11. 12. 13. 14. 15. 16. 17. 18. 19. 20. 21. 22.

CHAPTER 6

1. 2. 3. 4. 5. 6. 7. 8. 9. 10. 11. 12. 13. 14. 15. 16. 17. 18. 19. 20. 21. 22. 23. 24. 25. 26. 27.

28. 29. 30. 31. 32. 33. 34. 35. 36. 37. 38. 39. 40. 41. 42. 43. 44. 45. 46. 47. 48. 49. 50.

CHAPTER 7

1. 2. 3. 4. 5. 6. 7. 8. 9. 10. 11. 12. 13. 14. 15. 16. 17. 18. 19. 20. 21. 22. 23. 24. 25. 26. 27. 28.

29. 30. 31. 32. 33. 34. 35. 36. 37. 38. 39. 40. 41. 42. 43. 44. 45. 46. 47. 48. 49. 50. 51. 52. 53. 54. 55. 56. 57. 58. 59. 60. 61. 62. 63. 64. 65. 66. 67.

CHAPTER 8

1. 2. 3. 4. 5. 6. 7. 8. 9. 10. 11. 12.

13. 14. 15. 16. 17. 18. 19. 20. 21. 22. 23. 24. 25. 26. 27. 28. 29. 30. 31.

CHAPTER 9

1. 2. 3. 4. 5. 6. 7. 8. 9. 10. 11. 12. 13. 14. 15. 16. 17. 18. 19. 20. 21. 22. 23. 24. 25. 26. 27. 28. 29. 30. 31. 32.